Certified Nurse Educator Review Book

The Official NLN Guide to the CNE Exam

Certified Nurse Educator Review Book

The Official NLN Guide to the CNE Exam

Edited by

Linda Caputi, EdD, RN, CNE, ANEF

National League
for **Nursing**

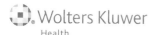
. Wolters Kluwer
Health

Philadelphia · Baltimore · New York · London
Buenos Aires · Hong Kong · Sydney · Tokyo

Acquisitions Editor: Sherry Dickinson
Product Development Editor: Meredith L. Brittain
Production Project Manager: Joan Sinclair
Designer: Holly McLaughlin
Illustration: Jennifer Clements
Manufacturing Coordinator: Karin Duffield
Composition: Aptara, Inc.

351 West Camden Street   Two Commerce Square/2001 Market Street
Baltimore, MD 21201   Philadelphia, PA 19103

Printed in the United States

ISBN 978-1-934758-20-5

Library of Congress Cataloging-in-Publication Data

Certified nurse educator review book : the official NLN guide to the CNE exam / edited by Linda Caputi.
    p. ; cm.
Includes bibliographical references and index.
ISBN 978-1-934758-20-5 (alk. paper)
I. Caputi, Linda, editor of compilation. II. National League for Nursing, issuing body.
[DNLM: 1. Faculty, Nursing—United States—Problems and Exercises. 2. Certification—United States. 3. Education, Nursing—methods—United States—Problems and Exercises. 4. Teaching—methods—United States—Problems and Exercises. WY 18.2]
RT90
610.73071′1—dc23
                                                                                2014001448

Disclaimer
Care has been taken to confirm the accuracy of the information presented and to describe generally accepted practices. However, the authors, editors, and publisher are not responsible for errors or omissions or for any consequences from application of the information in this book and make no warranty, expressed or implied, with respect to the currency, completeness, or accuracy of the contents of the publication. Application of this information in a particular situation remains the professional responsibility of the practitioner; the clinical treatments described and recommended may not be considered absolute and universal recommendations.

The authors, editors, and publisher have exerted every effort to ensure that drug selection and dosages set forth in this text are in accordance with the current recommendations and practice at the time of publication. However, in view of ongoing research, changes in government regulations, and the constant flow of information relating to drug therapy and drug reactions, the reader is urged to check the package insert for each drug for any change in indications and dosages and for added warnings and precautions. This is particularly important when the recommended agent is a new or infrequently employed drug.

Some drugs and medical devices presented in this publication have Food and Drug Administration (FDA) clearance for limited use in restricted research settings. It is the responsibility of the health care provider to ascertain the FDA status of each drug or device planned for use in his or her clinical practice.

To purchase additional copies of this book, call our customer service department at (800) 638-3030 or fax orders to (301) 223-2320. International customers should call (301) 223-2300. Visit Wolters Kluwer Health | Lippincott Williams & Wilkins online at www.lww.com. Visit the National League for Nursing online at www.nln.org.

DRC1217

About the Editor

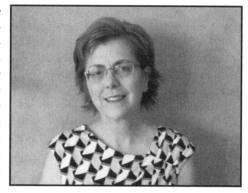

Linda Caputi, EdD, RN, CNE, ANEF, is the editor of the "Innovation Center," a column in the National League for Nursing's journal *Nursing Education Perspectives*. She is a certified nurse educator and a fellow in the NLN's Academy of Nursing Education. She is professor emerita, College of DuPage, and most currently taught in an online master's in nursing education program. She has won six awards for teaching excellence from Sigma Theta Tau and is included in three different years in the *Who's Who Among America's Teachers*. The second edition of her book *Teaching Nursing: The Art and Science* was selected as the winner of the 2010 Top Teaching Tools Award in the print category from the *Journal of Nursing Education*. She has recently completed a three-year term on the NLN's Board of Governors.

She is also president of Linda Caputi, Inc., a nursing education consulting company, and has worked with hundreds of nursing programs over the past 20 years on topics related to revising curriculum, transforming clinical education, test-item writing, and test construction, using an evidence-based model for NCLEX® success, assisting with accreditation, and numerous other nursing education topics.

About the Contributors

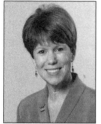

Gail Baumlein, PhD, RN, CNS, CNE, ANEF, has been a nurse for more than 30 years, with more than 20 years in academia. Her practice areas include pediatrics, emergency nursing, and adult health. She has held faculty and leadership positions in schools, colleges, and universities and has been involved in development and implementation of numerous new programs and colleges. She has worked in many areas of nursing education, including diploma, associate's degree, BSN, MSN, and DNP programs. She has also had the opportunity to be involved in faculty development and mentoring with many nurse educators across the country, focusing on technology in education and active teaching and learning strategies in the classroom, clinical, and online settings. Her research has focused on online education, faculty mentoring, and educational assessment and evaluation. She has been honored to be selected as the University of Akron College of Nursing's distinguished alumni and to be inducted as a fellow to the Academy of Nursing Education. She serves as governor at large on the National League for Nursing Board of Governors.

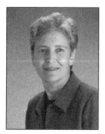

Wanda Blaser Bonnel, PhD, RN, GNP-BC, ANEF, is an associate professor at the University of Kansas School of Nursing. As a specialist in geriatrics and nursing education, she teaches courses in the master's, DNP, and PhD programs. She is a fellow in the National League for Nursing Academy and a recent recipient of the Chancellor's Distinguished Teaching Award at the University of Kansas. She has had leadership for multiple funded grants, including the ongoing Health Professions Educator Certificate. She has published numerous peer reviewed abstracts and articles in her geriatric and educator specialties. Her two coauthored texts, *Teaching Technologies in Nursing and the Health Professions* and *Proposal Writing for Nursing Capstones and Clinical Project,* help prepare future nursing professionals for the changing world of health care.

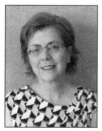

Linda Caputi, EdD, RN, CNE, ANEF, is the editor of the "Innovation Center," a column in the National League for Nursing's journal *Nursing Education Perspectives.* She is a certified nurse educator and a fellow in the NLN's Academy of Nursing Education. She is professor emerita, College of DuPage, and most currently taught in an online master's in nursing education program. She has won six awards for teaching excellence from Sigma Theta Tau and is included in three different years in the *Who's Who Among America's Teachers.* The second edition of her book *Teaching Nursing: The Art and Science* was selected as the winner of the 2010 Top Teaching Tools Award in the print category from the *Journal of Nursing Education.* She has recently completed a three-year term on the NLN's Board of Governors. She is also president of Linda

Caputi, Inc., a nursing education consulting company, and has worked with hundreds of nursing programs over the past 20 years on topics related to revising curriculum, transforming clinical education, test-item writing, and test construction, using an evidence-based model for NCLEX® success, assisting with accreditation, and numerous other nursing education topics.

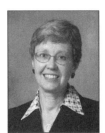

Marilyn Frenn, PhD, RN, CNE, FTOS, ANEF, has published studies related to teaching excellence and worked with PhD students on cultural aspects related to success in nursing school and as a new graduate. She currently serves on the National League for Nursing (NLN) Board of Governors. She is a former chair of the Nursing Education Research Advisory Council of the NLN and the Midwest Nursing Research Society's Nursing Education Research Section, former president of the Wisconsin League for Nursing, and was honored with an Outstanding Leadership Award from the NLN Constituent Advisory Council. She teaches the Nursing Education Research, Policy, and Leadership course in the PhD program at Marquette University College of Nursing and the graduate research course. She completed a postdoctoral research fellowship at the University of Michigan related to her research in obesity prevention and amelioration.

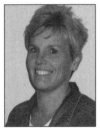

Susan Luparell, PhD, CNS-BC, CNE, is an associate professor at Montana State University, where she has been involved in both the baccalaureate and graduate nursing programs since 1997. She has been an active participant in the curriculum development of both programs, having served as a longtime member, as well as chairperson, of the curriculum committee. Additionally, she is a seasoned instructor who has received multiple commendations over the years for excellence in teaching. She is an expert on the dynamics between teacher and learner in nursing education and their influence on the processes of teaching and learning. She is a nationally recognized speaker and author on the topic of incivility in nursing education and has authored chapters on this topic in several leading nursing education textbooks. Her scholarship focuses on the ethical implications of incivility, including how it affects others and how it can be managed in academic as well as in clinical settings. Her clinical expertise is in adult cardiovascular and critical care nursing. Prior to moving into academia, she practiced as a clinical nurse specialist in the acute care setting. She maintains a per diem position at the local hospital, where she continues to practice at the bedside.

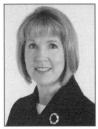

Jan M. Nick, PhD, RNC-OB, CNE, ANEF, holds dual appointments at Loma Linda University, California, and Saniku Gakuin College, Japan. At LLU, she directs and teaches in the Pipeline Program for a Diverse Nursing Workforce, a program for underrepresented or underprivileged students applying to the nursing program. In Japan, she has been the dean of the nursing department since March 2013. She has developed expertise with technology as a tool for the learner-centered approach to teaching and uses the team-based learning (TBL) approach. For the past six years she has served on the National League for Nursing (NLN) Academic Nurse Certification Commission, and she is a newly appointed member of the NLN INESA Global Taskforce.

She was a Fulbright scholar to Paraguay where she worked with the National University of Asunción School of Nursing and introduced Spanish open access resources to help them achieve evidence-based information competency. Her research interests include open access of scholarly information, distance mentoring, and evidence-based practice, and she travels the globe giving presentations to nursing faculty on these topics.

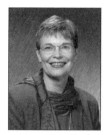

Nancy C. Sharts-Hopko, PhD, RN, CNE, FAAN, is a professor in the College of Nursing at Villanova University and director of the doctoral program. In the mid-1980s she lived for most of three years in Asia, where she served as a short-term consultant for the World Health Organization in Bangladesh and taught and conducted research at St. Luke's College of Nursing, Tokyo. Her research has focused on women's perceived well-being and related factors during life and health transitions, and her current research focuses on health issues related to low vision. With a background in maternal-infant and women's health nursing, she served on the Food and Drug Administration's (FDA) Advisory Committee on Maternal Health and Fertility Drugs from 1992 to 1995 and was a member of the FDA's Advisory Committee on Obstetrical and Gynecological Devices from 1999 to 2003. Since its inception through 2011, she has served as a member and chair of the National League for Nursing Certification Commission. She serves as treasurer of the Board of Sigma Theta Tau International, and she is a fellow in the American Academy of Nursing.

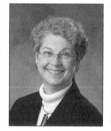

Theresa M. "Terry" Valiga, EdD, RN, CNE, FAAN, ANEF, is a professor and director of the Institute for Educational Excellence at the Duke University School of Nursing (Durham, North Carolina). Immediately prior to her appointment at Duke, she served as the chief program officer at the National League for Nursing; prior to that, she served on the faculty and held administrative positions in five universities over a 26-year period: Trenton State College (in New Jersey), Seton Hall University (in New Jersey), Georgetown University (in Washington, D.C.), Villanova University (in Pennsylvania), and Fairfield University (in Connecticut), where she was the dean of the School of Nursing for four years. She has completed research related to student learning, curriculum design, and leadership development and has received grants to support her scholarly endeavors. She has published extensively on a variety of leadership and education-related topics and has coauthored five books, one on each of the following topics: the nurse educator in academe; using the arts and humanities to teach nursing; clinical nursing education; achieving excellence in nursing education; and leadership (the latter in its fourth edition). In addition, she has presented papers and workshops at national and international conferences and served as a consultant to many schools of nursing throughout the United States, as well as in Canada, Japan, Bermuda, and China. Additionally, she has provided leadership in several professional organizations, including service on national governing boards. In recognition of her sustained contributions to nursing scholarship and nursing education, she has received several prestigious national awards and been inducted into the Academy of Nursing Education and the American Academy of Nursing.

Foreword

Edited by Dr. Linda Caputi, EdD, RN, CNE, ANEF, *Certified Nurse Educator Review Book: The Official NLN Guide to the CNE Exam* is a thorough, well-organized resource for nurse educators who aspire to have their knowledge and expertise acknowledged.

The National League for Nursing's (NLN) Certified Nurse Educator (CNE) credential is the only official recognition of "excellence in the advanced specialty role of the academic nurse educator." The program was initiated in 2005, one of the NLN's groundbreaking initiatives to recognize excellence and innovation. Now in its eighth year, the CNE program has been a resounding success. More than 4,000 nurse educators in all 50 states hold the CNE credential, and the program continues to enjoy a high level of recertifications.

To support applicants' preparation for the rigor of the exam, the CNE program has provided the *CNE Candidate Handbook*, self-assessment exams, and an ongoing series of continuing education workshops.

Now, in *Certified Nurse Educator Review Book: The Official NLN Guide to the CNE Exam*, Dr. Caputi supplements these resources with a user-friendly, yet scholarly, resource. A renowned provider of continuing education for nurse educators, Dr. Caputi exemplifies excellence and innovation. A CNE and a fellow in the NLN's Academy of Nursing Education, Dr. Caputi has a long history of commitment to advancing the mission and goals of the NLN: presenting at NLN education summits and serving as a member of the Board of Governors, the NLN Think Tank for Transforming Clinical Education, the NLN Nursing Education Research and Advisory Council, and the Electronic Repository Task Force. The author of a number of well-received books on nursing education, Dr. Caputi edited *Innovations in Nursing Education: Building the Future of Nursing* (2013), which was recently published by the NLN and Wolters Kluwer Health. She is professor emerita at the College of DuPage in Glen Ellyn, Illinois, and has more than 25 years of teaching experience.

This book includes a chapter for each of the eight Core Competencies of Academic Nurse Educators that appear on the CNE test blueprint. Each chapter includes the related task statements; incorporates an in-depth, scholarly description of the competency and relevant research; and is followed by practice questions. Faculty using this official NLN guide to prepare for the CNE exam will find cutting-edge theory and evidence-based knowledge and strategies designed to help them move forward in achieving the CNE credential.

Deborah Lindell, DNP, RN, CNE, ANEF
Director, Graduate Entry Nursing Program
Frances Payne Bolton School of Nursing
Case Western Reserve University
Cleveland, Ohio

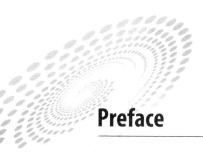

Preface

Welcome to *Certified Nurse Educator Review Book: The Official NLN Guide to the CNE Exam*! The National League for Nursing is delighted to provide this resource for nurse educators. The purpose of this book is to provide an overall review in preparation for taking the CNE examination and is based on the CNE examination test blueprint. Therefore, this book is intended to provide the type of information that relates to each category on the test blueprint.

Book Organization

The book is divided into chapters—one chapter for each of the eight categories on the test blueprint. Each chapter provides an overview of the content included on the CNE exam blueprint.

Please note it is not an exhaustive discussion of all possible topics that may appear on the examination. As those who have taken a certification examination in nursing know, it would be difficult, if not impossible, to completely cover all possible information related to each of the areas of the CNE test blueprint. However, this book presents the major categories, then provides the readers with concrete information to guide their study.

Each chapter provides practice test items. These test items were developed by item writers for the actual CNE examination, thereby providing an accurate reflection of the types of questions you will encounter on the examination.

Studying for the Exam

A common question asked by attendees of a CNE review course is, "How should I study for the exam?" One approach is the following:

1. Review the CNE eligibility requirements (available online at www.nln.org).
2. Read the current *CNE Candidate Handbook* (available online at www.nln.org).
3. Set a target date for taking the CNE examination.
4. Review this book.
5. Develop a list of topics with which you are unfamiliar or consider areas in which you need further study.
6. Develop a calendar of study.
7. Consult the publications listed in the *CNE Candidate Handbook* and review the areas you identified as needing further study.
8. Take NLN's self-assessment examination (SAE), which is available for purchase at www.nln.org/certification/information/sae.htm. The Internet-based SAE is half the length of the actual examination and provides practice for taking CNE-type questions written by CNE item writers. Rationales for correct and incorrect answers are provided.
9. Based on your results on the SAE, determine areas in which you may need additional study.

10. Review the identified areas for further study using this book as well as other publications listed in the *CNE Candidate Handbook*.
11. Optional: Attend a CNE review course. You can find information about CNE review courses on the NLN website.
12. Take the CNE examination.

It is helpful to recognize your individual preferences for study. Whereas some candidates prefer to study alone, others find forming a study group with other faculty very helpful. A convenient way to form a group is to work with faculty within your own school. Groups can meet in the workplace over lunch or another time convenient for the faculty.

Certification as a Mark of Distinction

Taking the CNE examination is an exciting adventure. Certification is a mark of professionalism. Certification as a nurse educator is a mark of distinction for nursing faculty and recognition of the advanced specialty role of the academic nurse educator. Best wishes as you embark on this excellence initiative offered by the National League for Nursing.

Acknowledgments

I here acknowledge the many people who worked tirelessly over the past decade to make the Certified Nurse Educator (CNE) program a reality. As explained by Dr. Ortelli (2010), the NLN engaged in a series of tasks that culminated in the current CNE examination. These tasks included:

- A think tank in 2001
- A position statement, "Preparation of Nurse Educators," issued by the NLN Board of Governors in 2002
- A feasibility study or needs assessment in 2003, which revealed that 80 percent of deans and directors saw certification of nurse educators as beneficial to their programs
- A task group on nurse educator competencies, which developed the core competencies of nurse educators
- Completion of a task analysis to provide content validity to the certification examination
- Development of the test blueprint
- Development of the examination

The above tasks brought the test to nurse educators for the first time in September 2005. Since 2005, thousands of nurse educators have taken the examination and are now certified. These early efforts built a strong foundation on which the NLN continues this important work.

I thank Dr. Nancy Sharts-Hopko for reviewing all the end-of-chapter practice test items. Dr. Sharts-Hopko offered her expert review of these test items, for which I am extremely grateful.

I thank all the chapter authors. As the editor, I understand the quality of this book is a direct expression of the work of the chapter authors. Each author represents nursing education at its very best; I am very grateful for the time and expertise they unselfishly shared to make this book a reality.

Finally, I am grateful for the time and work of Dr. Elaine Tagliareni and Dr. Linda Christensen of the National League for Nursing. These colleagues provide the behind-the-scenes administrative work for much of what we enjoy from the NLN. I appreciate the patience and professionalism they provided during all our interactions.

Reference

Ortelli, T. (2010). The certified nurse educator credential. In L. Caputi (Ed.), *Teaching nursing: The art and science* (pp. 564–585). Glen Ellyn, IL: DuPage Press.

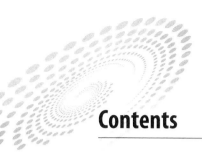

Contents

Facilitate Learning

Jan M. Nick, PhD, RNC-OB, CNE, ANEF

The CNE Test Plan Lists the Following for the Area of Facilitate Learning:

1. Facilitate Learning
  A. Implement a variety of teaching strategies appropriate to:
  1. content
  2. setting (i.e., clinical versus classroom)
  3. learner needs
  4. learning style
  5. desired learner outcomes
  6. method of delivery (e.g., face-to-face, remote, simulation)
  B. Use teaching strategies based on:
  1. educational theory
  2. evidence-based practices related to education
  C. Modify teaching strategies and learning experiences based on consideration of learners':
  1. cultural background
  2. past clinical experiences
  3. past educational and life experiences
  4. generational groups (i.e., age)
  D. Use information technologies to support the teaching-learning process
  E. Practice skilled oral and written (including electronic) communication that reflects an awareness of self and relationships with learners (e.g., evaluation, mentorship, and supervision)
  F. Communicate effectively orally and in writing with an ability to convey ideas in a variety of contexts
  G. Model reflective thinking practices, including critical thinking
  H. Create opportunities for learners to develop their own critical thinking skills
  I. Create a positive learning environment that fosters a free exchange of ideas
  J. Show enthusiasm for teaching, learning, and the nursing profession that inspires and motivates students
  K. Demonstrate personal attributes that facilitate learning (e.g., caring, confidence, patience, integrity, respect, and flexibility)
  L. Respond effectively to unexpected events that affect instruction
  M. Develop collegial working relationships with clinical agency personnel to promote positive learning environments
  N. Use knowledge of evidence-based practice to instruct learners
  O. Demonstrates ability to teach clinical skills
  P. Act as a role model in practice settings
  Q. Foster a safe learning environment

This chapter focuses on competencies and best practices for creating a learning environment in the academic setting. Examples of research are cited to provide direction for specific issues in nursing education. This chapter focuses on strategies nurse educators use to maximize many of the variables that affect student learning, so that students can reach their full career potential.

IMPLEMENT A VARIETY OF TEACHING STRATEGIES

The nurse educator has a responsibility to create optimal learning conditions. This requires multiple approaches to deliver accurate and appropriate learning in a variety of contexts to meet the learner's needs and achieve desired outcomes. Effective teachers use active student learning techniques, demonstrate enthusiasm, provide diverse opportunities to learn, integrate concepts and ideas into their courses, promote critical questioning, and give timely feedback to students' responses (Zurmehly & Leadingham, 2008).

Learner Needs

With a student-centered model of education, the teacher is responsible for creating different learning strategies to meet the varied needs of students. When learning environments are tailored to student needs, improved outcomes occur and course failures are minimized. Although needs may be myriad, the skilled nurse educator knows how to incorporate active learning strategies, technology, and different learning styles so students are invited to participate in the learning process.

Active Learning

Students learn better if they are actively engaged in the learning activity. Professional organizations such as the American Association of Colleges of Nursing (2009) and the National League for Nursing (2006) also support this approach. During face-to-face learning encounters, faculty traditionally use lengthy periods of lecture and focus on conveying content, leaving little time for application, analysis, evaluation, and synthesis. National survey data demonstrate that nursing students do not identify active learning strategies being used in their classes (Popkess & McDaniel, 2011). Myriad activities that shift the focus from the teacher toward the student can be used in the classroom and are supported by research. Examples include unfolding case scenarios (Benner, Sutphen, Leonard, & Day, 2010), practice testing (DuHamel et al., 2011), role playing (Levitt & Adelman, 2010), and audience response clickers (discussed in another section). Activities, often rooted in a technology-rich environment, ask the student to engage in decision-making about information and support the learning process.

Technology-Rich Environment

Students come from a technology-rich environment, and when faculty use media and technology in the learning session, students respond favorably (Jones, Henderson, & Sealover, 2009). Wiki technology is an excellent strategy to have students practice collaboration skills; it can also be used for writing assignments (Collier, 2010) and for sharing information, resources, and experiences (Kardong-Edgren et al., 2009). Learning management systems now have built-in wiki features or students can use Google Docs®. Tweeting, used as a teaching strategy, began in 2008 in the nursing literature. A Tweet is a post of 140 characters or less, making it an efficient form of distilling information to the most important elements. Trueman and Miles (2011) used this Web 2.0 strategy to help student groups present essential information about an assigned health topic. Students worked in pairs and took one aspect of the nursing process. Each topic had five pairs of students. The whole group validated each other's Tweets before presenting to the whole class. The authors concluded that using a technology-based process grounded in the social context of collaborative learning helped students absorb information.

Lancaster, Wong, and Roberts (2012) studied the effect of blending technology into the classroom by having students listen to taped didactic materials prior to class. This left time for in-class application and discussion. Results showed significant improvement in test scores because students could apply material, and they rated this technology-infused technique as helpful in supporting their learning.

Using Learning Styles   *These have been disproven!*

The term *learning style* is broadly used in the literature to refer to learners' classification schemes when engaged in learning, depending on their dominating cognitive and psychological traits (Kyprianidou, Demetriadis, Tsiatsos, & Pombortsis, 2012). Tailoring activities to learning styles so students' natural dominant traits can be used will actually allow them to learn better (Rundle & Dunn, 2008).

Perceptual learning styles involve using the auditory, visual, auditory–verbal, tactile, and kinesthetic senses to gain information about the given environment or situation (Rundle & Dunn, 2008). Examples of incorporating learning styles into course assignments could include:

- Having visual learners draw information to show how concepts fit together, such as concept maps, and then post the work to a course website.
- Having students audiotape explanations and post them to a course website. Auditory–verbal learners learn best when given the opportunity to discuss new material, so they can make information personally meaningful. These auditory–verbal learners would likely learn while constructing and taping the work, and auditory learners would be relistening to materials that would help them learn. These activities would support both types of learning styles.
- Creating experiences where tactile learners can use fine motor skills, such as typing summaries and posting on a class wiki, which would solidify their learning. Both tactile and kinesthetic learners prefer a hands-on approach. Kinesthetic learners learn best when asked to re-create information using their gross motor skills (i.e., have them prepare a demonstration for the whole class).

Because learning styles are not static and can change over time (Cools, Evans, & Redmond, 2009), teachers should help students become aware of their learning styles and plan reinventory sessions throughout the nursing curriculum. Not only would knowledge of this be helpful to students, but students' awareness and appreciation of different learning styles would be enhanced, bringing increased value and understanding of teammates (Kyprianidou et al., 2012).

Knowledge of learning styles can also be applied to other situations in the learning environment. Kyprianidou et al. (2012) discovered that using learning styles to assign groups at the beginning of the term was an efficient way to increase team functioning when groups comprised students from each learning style. Nurse educators desiring to increase their competency in meeting learner needs will put into practice those activities that support diverse learning styles.

Desired Learner Outcomes   *Outcomes = Know, do, value*

KSA

Learning outcomes should be student focused and clearly articulate what students should know (knowledge), be able to do (skills), and value (attitude) (Billings, 2012). These student-centered outcomes are intended to inform students about the expectations they must meet. Assignments should directly align to course student learning outcomes and be clearly demonstrated in the course syllabus. Topic or module objectives should be clearly linked to course, program, and institutional student learning outcomes. Student learning outcomes need to be constructed for each learning event, regardless of the setting, clinical emphasis, or program level. They can also be used to focus instruction, create test blueprints, generate test items, and evaluate student progression. Nursing faculty are excellent at planning individual class objectives and staying on point. By creating summary tables or concept maps of how assignments, topic objectives, and course student learning outcomes help achieve program and institutional learning outcomes as well as meet requirements of regional and professional accrediting bodies, faculty are being intentional about the larger context of the learning environment and demonstrating how all levels of the curriculum are congruent.

Determining Appropriate Content

When planning content to be incorporated within the learning environment, how does the nurse educator determine best practice? What topics should the educator include and how broadly or deeply should the content be covered? Faculty often use five avenues to determine appropriateness of topics, breadth, and depth: (a) personal opinion, experience, or tradition, (b) course textbooks, (c) professional accrediting bodies, (d) professional clinical organizations, and (e) national licensure and certification councils. The first method creates inappropriate variation in the curriculum and is not supported by evidence; the second tempts faculty to try to cover all the topics included in the book, thus encouraging the ever-expanding course curriculum. The third avenue, professional accrediting bodies, sets standards and competencies that nursing programs must meet, therefore, faculty must include that required content to receive accreditation. The fourth, professional clinical organizations, provides emerging evidence during conventions and conferences, through publications and guidelines, and is a valuable asset to use. The fifth resource, national licensure and certification councils, provides reliable and valid information based on evidence collected from practice analyses or role delineation research. The nurse educator monitors the national licensure and certification council websites for updated information on the conceptual structure of the exam, question format, and content. By doing so, faculty use evidence to make decisions about content depth and breadth, thus upholding the evidence-based practice of nursing education.

Faculty recognize the state of excessive, additive, or obese curricular content (Giddens & Brady, 2007; Ironside, 2004; Tanner, 2004). But faculty also continue to focus on teaching content (Benner et al., 2010). Because of this, many authors have implored that nursing education make a paradigm shift from the heavy content-laden body system approach toward a conceptually based curriculum that will help students learn the material better and provide more opportunities to determine appropriate action in clinical situations (Benner et al., 2010; Dalley, Candela, & Benzel-Lindley, 2008; Giddens & Brady, 2007; Giddens et al., 2008). The Institute of Medicine has recognized the expanding curricular content and has recommended changing the emphasis to testing competencies and teaching students how to adapt to new models of care and ever-changing science and patient demographics (IOM, 2011, p. 172). Given the conceptual organization of national licensing and certification exams, this recommendation is germane for today's curriculum. In addition, shifting to a conceptually based model of teaching would support deep learning, because students tend to get lost in details and forget facts when content is stressed over concepts.

Setting and Method of Delivery

A variety of settings and contexts for the learning session are available to create the learning experience. Students can experience instruction using face-to-face, hybrid, online, clinical, and simulation environments. Each context has its own best practices and requires intentional action to facilitate student learning.

Face-to-Face Context

The traditional face-to-face method for teaching has transitioned to a hybrid combination of face-to-face interaction with augmented online presence. Uploading documents, articles, audio clips and videos, and quizzes is now possible with Learning Management Systems, which allow the student to learn anywhere, anytime. Research, however, shows that students still value the face-to-face environment for the realism, immediacy of feedback, and human connectedness it offers (Gruendemann, 2011). Face-to-face learning, however, is not necessarily the preferred context in which to learn. Wells and Dellinger (2011) tested three types of settings (face-to-face, online, or using compressed video offsite to attend classes at the host site) and found the learning environment was not as important as the quality of instruction. In addition, there was no difference in perceived learning, feelings of connectedness, and interactions between learner–learner and learner–instructor methods.

Online Context

Online education has been a significant part of the teaching–learning landscape since 1991, and the expectations for meeting the same academic standards exist for both online education and face-to-face instruction. It is important to keep in mind that technology should never overshadow the intent of teaching students.

Best practices in online education include sufficient orientation to the technology, appropriate time allotted, timeliness of feedback, appropriate use of technology, and faculty–student and student–student interactions (Seiler & Billings, 2004). Timely feedback to students is another best practice, as the immediacy helps students learn. By waiting too long to provide feedback, students have moved their attention to other learning matters, assignments, and exam preparations and a learning moment is lost.

Students like online learning because it offers the convenience of learning at their own pace and eliminates or decreases driving distance to the campus (Wells & Dellinger, 2011). It also provides anonymity and voice to introverted students and decreases the distractions found in the classroom (Reilly, Gallagher-Lepak, & Killion, 2012). Educators must acknowledge the potential isolation or loneliness students can experience (Reilly et al., 2012). Establishing community early on has been shown to be the most effective strategy to improve learning, increase retention, and combat loneliness (Gallagher-Lepak, Reilly, & Killion, 2009).

Clinical Context

Nurse educators often struggle with determining clinical competence or incompetence or whether the student is just trying to master the particular clinical subject matter. Students and faculty recognize subjectivity can be a factor in determining competence. Lewallen and DeBrew (2012) provided evidence to help faculty answer this question. During the interviews of 24 experienced nurse faculty, themes emerged describing successful characteristics of nursing students in clinical settings: (a) coming prepared for the clinical experience, (b) demonstrating the ability to think critically, (c) communicating effectively with faculty, staff, patients, and peers, and (d) having a positive attitude toward learning, showing progress, and accepting feedback. Characteristics that indicate a student should fail a clinical would be the opposite of these themes as well as if students jeopardize patient safety or commit legal or ethical violations. Additionally, students must also meet expectations for all course student learning outcomes as identified on the clinical evaluation tool. It is heartening that these characteristics in their positive aspects align nicely with professional nursing education expectations of critical thinking, communication, teamwork, safety, and lifelong learning. Tanicala, Scheffer, and Roberts (2011) conducted focus group interviews with 11 faculty from a variety of public and private universities teaching in different levels in nursing education. Five themes arose: (a) safety issues, (b) inability to think critically, (c) unethical behavior, (d) inability to communicate effectively, and (e) inability to meet course and agency standards. The authors constructed a detailed model with various subthemes under each category that give definitive direction to faculty who have to determine whether to pass or fail a student in clinical practice based on these characteristics. There is striking concordance among all the authors' conclusions. However, these characteristics should be inherent in the behavioral expectations as noted on the clinical evaluation tool.

Faculty must be tenacious about helping students with learning prioritization skills because this activity will help them develop clinical expertise (Benner et al., 2010; Lake, Moss, & Duke, 2009). Benner et al. (2010, p. 50) emphasized students needing the ability to develop clinical judgment through coaching on priority setting in the context of multiple patient problems; they also encourage faculty to help students realize that priorities are in constant flux. Because additional health conditions can surface or unfold throughout the day, students must be able to reprioritize. Importantly, prioritization and delegation comprise the largest categories of questions tested on the NCLEX-RN® (National Council Licensure Examination for Registered Nurses)—almost one-quarter of all the questions on the exam are from these categories (National Council of State Boards of Nursing, 2012). Unfortunately, there seems to be a lack of formal instruction about prioritizing in either nursing curricula (Benner et al., 2010, p. 52) or popular nursing textbooks (Lake et al., 2009). These results have grave implications for educators. There is a stand-alone resource available for students to formally learn prioritization and delegation skills using case scenarios and NCLEX-style questions (LaCharity, Kumagai, & Bartz, 2013). Given that (a) nursing students need prioritization skills for clinical competence, (b) many nursing textbooks do not provide sections dedicated to the topic, and (c) the highest number of questions asked on the NCLEX is about prioritization and delegation, a best practice for faculty is to be very intentional about facilitating students' learning prioritization.

Some nursing schools and clinical agencies are partnering to create dedicated education units (DEUs). With this clinical model, health care units are dedicated to the instruction of students, and clinical nurses function as instructors, typically overseeing no more than two students at a time with six students to a unit; they are supported by a university faculty member who oversees the instruction (IOM, 2011, p. 190). Groups of two students work with each faculty member or clinical nurse instructor, thus providing opportunities for student-to-student peer collaboration as well as constant nurse-to-nursing student interaction. Moore and Nahigian (2013) compared nursing student perspectives between DEUs and traditional clinical learning units and found that students from DEUs rated collaboration between nurses and nursing student higher than students learning in traditional clinicals. Anecdotal comments by institutions indicate student learning is enhanced, and students believed they belonged and were considered part of the team (Tuohy, 2011). When Mulready-Shick, Kafel, and Banister (2009) interviewed 16 students who participated in a pilot DEU project, students identified experiencing increased learning about (a) teamwork and collaboration through cooperation and a welcoming attitude, (b) safety with medications due to the low instructor-to-student ratios, (c) informatics in the form of availability of resources and electronic health records when they worked alongside the instructor or clincal nurse, (d) patient-centered care as they witnessed positive role modeling when their nurse interacted with patients, and (e) evidence-based practice (EBP) and quality improvement through unit-based teaching–learning projects.

Simulation Context

Simulation has exploded on the teaching–learning scene and is considered standard in nursing curricula. As recently as 2010, 77 percent of 1,060 nursing programs surveyed nationally used medium-fidelity and high-fidelity simulators and substituted traditional clinical time with simulation (Hayden, 2010). Each state board of nursing sets standards for simulation experiences; faculty must check with their state board of nursing to determine how much clinical time can be replaced with simulation. Because of the technology involved, the startup for simulation laboratories requires significant fiscal and personnel resources. Halstead et al. (2011) reported on using a simulation consortium to manage these costs and showed this method was very cost-effective, helped promote development of nurse educators within the community, and provided an avenue for networking and collaboration. Students responded favorably to the simulation experience as well; they reported having the opportunity to practice skills, think critically and problem solve in a controlled environment, foster teamwork, and rehearse communication skills (Richardson, Gilmartin, & Fulmer, 2012).

Nurse researchers are currently testing models where simulation provides a significant portion of the clinical learning experience. For example, Richardson et al. (2012) offered a model where up to half (50 percent) of the clinical education experience was conducted in the context of simulation. Benefits realized from this model included (a) reducing the number of students needing to be supervised in the clinical area at any given time to six students per faculty, (b) increasing the number of students enrolled in the nursing program, and (c) providing more intensive and individualized learning experiences in the clinical area.

An unanticipated finding faculty must address is the experience of assigning the observer role to students in the simulation laboratory. Beischel (2013) and Richardson et al. (2012) reported that the nonactive roles such as students watching other students was the least helpful learning experience. However, assigning students as observer so they can learn from others' successes and mistakes is a common practice. By applying knowledge of learning styles, students who are either audio learners or visual learners could benefit from taking on the role of an observer, while auditory–verbal, tactile, and kinesthetic learners may not have the best learning experience. Research in this area is needed.

Faculty interested in meeting simulation best practice benchmarks can monitor key nursing education websites devoted specifically to simulation. The Simulation Information Resource Center (http://sirc.nln.org/) of the National League for Nursing and the International Nursing Association for Clinical Simulation and Learning (https://inacsl.org/) provide excellent resources.

USE TEACHING STRATEGIES BASED ON EDUCATIONAL THEORY AND EVIDENCE-BASED PRACTICES RELATED TO EDUCATION

Having knowledge of and reflecting on various educational theories help the nurse educator plan the most effective and efficient learning environment for the students. Being cognizant of various theories is a prerequisite to effective teaching (Candela, 2012). Because theory undergirds all activities, any of the educational theories can be used in a variety of settings and venues (e.g., face-to-face, online, graduate and undergraduate, didactic, and clinical). See Appendix A of this book for principles and application to learning for selected educational learning theories.

An excellent resource to use when learning about educational theory is pedagogical literature. Unfortunately, Patterson and Klein (2012) discovered very few nurse faculty (4 percent) used the Education Resources Information Center (ERIC) database, a primary database for educational research. By their very practice as educators, nurse faculty have a dual responsibility to continually immerse themselves in teaching–learning literature as well as clinical literature to provide relevant clinical information using evidence-based teaching methods.

Educational Theory

Best practices in teaching acknowledge the paradigm shift from a teacher-centered locus of responsibility to teach content (i.e., lecture format) toward a student-centered approach because the faculty-dominated classroom is not conducive to the development of critical thinking (Rowles, 2012; Seiler & Billings, 2004). In addition, an environment that focuses heavily on content delivery leaves very little time for higher-order thinking such as application, analysis, synthesis, and evaluation. Additionally, Seiler and Billings (2004) showed that students want to participate in active learning strategies. Any active learning technique that engages students and requires them to think critically supports deep learning (Mareno, Bremner, & Emerson, 2010); it also involves the learner in practicing the six learning domains proposed by Bloom, Engelhart, Furst, Hill, and Krathwohl (1956): knowledge, comprehension, application, analysis, synthesis, and evaluation.

Many of the active learning methods involve group work, higher-order critical thinking, problem solving, and self-initiated learning, all of which closely mirror the National League for Nursing's (2006) role competencies to think critically, communicate effectively, function as intra- and interdisciplinary member, and know how to find, manage, and use information and the American Association of Colleges of Nursing's (2009) competencies of collaboration, critical thinking, functioning as a part of a multidisciplinary team, and lifelong learning. Student-centered educational models produce greater student satisfaction, more student engagement, and higher scoring on examinations, whether in individual courses or collectively. When restructuring whole programs for active learning, use:

1. Competency-based or mastery learning (Roberts, Ingram, Flack, & Hayes, 2013)
2. Problem-based learning (PBL) (Baker, McDaniel, Pesut, & Fisher, 2007; Özbıçakçı, Bilik, & İntepeler, 2012)
3. Team-based learning (TBL) (Andersen, Strumpel, Fensom, & Andrews, 2011; Lubeck, Tschetter, & Mennenga, 2013; Sisk, 2011)

Evidence-Based Teaching Practices

In this age of EBP, the ethical and responsible approach for nurse educators is to ensure their practice of teaching is also evidence based. Although the concept of EBP is not new, as recently as a few years ago, Ferguson and Day (2005) postulated that EBP of nursing education was still a myth. Pennington and Spurlock (2010) systematically reviewed nursing education interventions for increasing NCLEX pass rates. They concluded that, of the studies focusing on student improvement, there was a lack of high-quality, randomized, controlled interventional studies. They also noted a paucity of interventional studies aimed at altering teacher-centered styles and improving faculty teaching styles.

Within the structure of student-centered models, faculty use a variety of embedded activities during the learning session that are firmly grounded in evidence. Some examples that engage students include (a) a technology-rich environment (discussed above), (b) collaborative testing, and (c) the use of response systems.

Collaborative Testing

Collaborative testing in nursing has been used to facilitate learning during testing, foster critical thinking in decision making, and improve group processing skills. Results, however, continue to be mixed. Sandahl (2010) tested two groups of nursing students and found higher scores with collaborative testing, yet this method did not significantly impact retention of course material as measured in the final exam. There were no differences in test scores between those who engaged in collaborative testing prior to the final and those who had not. Students, however, reported increased learning as a result of the collaboration. Wiggs (2010) had students take individual tests and then the collaborative test. Students liked collaborative testing because of their ability to apply critical thinking principles and to work as a team. The students, however, disliked the feeling of peer pressure from having to be prepared to defend answers. Centrella-Nigro (2012) found collaborative testing was an effective way to conduct posttest review—the majority of student questions were answered during the collaborative testing portion. In this study, the majority of students liked collaborating in a group and felt it enhanced their learning.

Response Systems

The master teacher seeks to engage students frequently during learning sessions with various activities. One example of a tool used for engaging the class is the student response system, also called a personal response system, audience response system, or classroom response system. These systems are used to poll students on a number of questions or to present multiple-choice questions for students to answer. The systems display the number of responses for each option. This active learning technique has been shown to be effective for engaging higher-level thinking and decision-making, providing immediate feedback for students, facilitating teacher–student communication, and helping faculty gauge student understanding (DeBourgh, 2008; Efstathiou & Bailey, 2012; Mareno et al., 2010; Revell & McCurry, 2010). Response systems can consist of dedicated electronic "clickers," cell phones, or paper-made response cards that are folded to show only one letter or number. Figure 1.1 shows how to make an ABCD response card out of paper. Companies such as Poll Everywhere (www. polleverywhere.com), mClk (www.mclkonline.com), and Mentimeter (www. mentimeter.com/audience-response-system) use text messaging technology as an audience response system, reducing the need to purchase hand-held audience response systems.

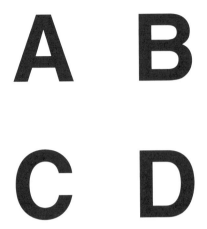

FIGURE 1.1 Example of a simple audience response system made out of a sheet of paper.

MODIFY TEACHING STRATEGIES AND LEARNING EXPERIENCES BASED ON CONSIDERATION OF LEARNERS' CHARACTERISTICS

A main goal of nursing education is to prepare students to meet diverse patients' needs. Accomplishing this goal can be met by increasing the diversity of nurses entering the workforce; however, the continued underrepresentation of racial and ethnic minority groups and men in nursing still exists (IOM, 2011, p. 164). This condition continues not because of noninterest on the part of the applicants—in fact, Burruss and Popkess (2012) speak of the applicant pools being more diverse. More men are entering the nursing profession, students may come from four different generational populations, and there is increased racial and ethnic diversity. The issue is, although a diverse student body enters nursing school, bias in the learning environment continues to exist, student success is not supported, and higher rates of attrition for these groups remain a factor.

Nurse educators must seek to eliminate any bias that interferes with student success. Recognizing biases and eliminating them require faculty to be self-reflective, flexible, creative, and intentional about offering different learning activities so a diverse group of students can succeed.

Multicultural Influences Affecting Learning

The American Association of Colleges of Nursing (2009) reported that one-fourth of all undergraduate and graduate nursing students represent minority groups. This statistic has not been fully realized until recently, because the proportion of racially and ethnically diverse nursing graduates has increased only gradually over the past two decades (HRSA, 2010).

With the move toward active learning, students with significant portions of their earlier education in different countries may not be socialized to the level of expected engagement and critical thinking. Often, students from some countries expect faculty to transmit all the knowledge, are taught to not raise questions, and are asked to memorize information (Amaro, Abriam-Yago, & Yoder, 2006). The passivity that may be present in these students is not evidence of disinterest, lack of knowledge, or indifference, but rather one of cultural clashing—students may believe it is inappropriate to speak up in class or to question authority. Orienting students to the educational model used in the course and the expectations for student participation hasten their socialization process and hence their success.

Another influence affecting learning is the inadvertent linguistic bias that can occur with multiple-choice questions (Bosher & Bowles, 2008; Lujan, 2008). Often, students recount that exam difficulty is not experienced with the content of multiple-choice questions but rather with the unnecessary complexity in the stem or options, grammatical errors, and lack of clarity or consistency in the use of words (Bosher & Bowles, 2008). Performing linguistic analysis and modification can eliminate bias yet maintain the integrity of the exam items.

Sentence completion items, irrelevant and unnecessary information, asking for priority actions without bolding or highlighting embedded or understood clauses, and unclear wording form the classic linguistic bias commonly found in multiple-choice questions (Bosher, 2009). Lampe and Tsaouse (2010) reviewed questions in a selected textbook publisher's test bank and found significant linguistic bias. One hundred percent of the questions were sentence completion format, priority questions did not use bolding or highlighting to emphasize important words, and 20 percent of the questions had embedded clauses. Students whose primary language is other than English have a difficult time determining the meaning of questions when the questions are biased toward students with a primary language of English.

Creating multiple-choice questions without linguistic bias takes commitment and intentionality by nurse educators. Course faculty can work collaboratively to create, review, and revise questions, or this can be accomplished at the departmental level by creating exam committees.

Generational Influences Affecting Learning

Because of differing life experiences for differing age groups, generational diversity is present. It is therefore imperative that nurse educators recognize that generational differences can explain part of the tension that potentially arises in the classroom when today's students act differently from yesterday's students. For faculty to be intentional about creating appropriate learning experiences for different generations, the nursing department should profile their student population.

Four primary groups of learners include (a) the traditionalists, (b) baby boomers, (c) Generation X, and (d) Generation Y (also known as millennials). The current mix of students in nursing school is primarily composed of those from Generations X and Y. These students are digital natives who prefer to use technology when learning (Godwin-Jones, 2005), like to create content on the web (Skiba, 2007), and are efficient multitaskers. Because of their ability to multitask, these students may need extra guidance in prioritizing activities (Burruss & Popkess, 2012). Asking Generation X and Generation Y students to sit and listen to a lecture is extremely difficult for them—they will attempt to do other activities while listening to a lecture. Two excellent resources summarizing the literature on generational abilities of different learners are Burruss and Popkess (2012) and Gibson (2009).

Gender Influences Affecting Learning

The growing body of literature on gender bias continues to remind nurse faculty there is still much to do to create an inclusive society. Although other health professions now experience gender parity, the nursing profession continues to lag significantly behind, as men compose just 7 percent of the nursing workforce (HRSA, 2010). Unfortunately, nurse educators continue to create an environment where male nursing students experience subtle bias cues (Meadus & Twomey, 2011). This may result in male nursing students continuing to experience higher attrition rates (McLaughlin, Muldoon, & Moutray, 2010; Pryjmachuk, Easton, & Littlewood, 2009). Unfortunately, findings also indicated that male students who do complete and graduate from nursing left with the impression that nursing was more appropriate for women than men (McLaughlin et al., 2010). The nursing literature continues to document the existence of gender bias, yet interventional research is scarce. Nursing as a profession urgently needs to test interventions to eradicate gender bias, so the profession will attract more men.

Past Clinical Experiences and Educational and Life Experiences

Becoming familiar with students' previous life experiences and helping them relate those experiences to their learning reinforce concepts and create deep learning (Knowles, 1980). Ramsden (2013) has been studying about teaching in the classroom for decades and asserted that the deepest roots and the strongest hold on how students interpret information are their prior understandings and life experiences. Master educators must use this information to their advantage. By getting to know students on a personal level in the educational setting, faculty can begin to understand the challenges that students face, the approaches they use, and the socialization needed to increase students' capacity for success. The combination of age, gender, race or ethnicity, and life experiences provides individuals with unique perspectives that contribute to the advancement of the nursing profession and better care for patients (IOM, 2011).

USE INFORMATION TECHNOLOGIES TO SUPPORT THE TEACHING–LEARNING PROCESS

The emergence of technology has created a whole new field of nursing informatics. The IOM predicts health informatics technology (HIT) will fundamentally change the way in which nurses plan, deliver, document, and review clinical care. Because nurses have the most sustained interactions with patients, they are often the greatest users of technology (IOM, 2011). Therefore, nurse educators must create opportunities for students to learn how to use HIT most effectively for improved patient care delivery.

Part of HIT is incorporating it into the teaching environment. Teaching students informatics literacy and using new types of evidence, or knowing how to find and display various health informatics media for online courses without infringing copyright, are skills faculty can use to facilitate learning. With the expansion of web-based courses in nursing education, faculty are faced with a greater responsibility to be copyright compliant (Dobbins, Souder, & Smith, 2005). Public domain videos, audio files, photos, and images can all be used for teaching purposes without worry of noncompliance. For copyrighted materials, faculty use either the Technology Education and Copyright Harmonization Act, the U.S. fair use guidelines, or the Common Creative Attributions License. The Technology Education and Copyright Harmonization Act allows faculty to use digital materials and upload to web pages intended for instruction; materials can remain on the web page for limited student use for two years (Lyons, 2010). The U.S. fair use guidelines are the most restrictive and prohibit users from copying and distributing without express permission from the copyright holder (U.S. Copyright Office, 2012). The Common Creative Attributions License is used with open access materials and allows users to download, copy, share, or use the work as long as they give attribution to the licensor (http://creativecommons.org/about/licenses).

The advent of evidence-based systematic reviews and clinical practice guidelines allows faculty choices about which evidence to use during the teaching–learning session and opens up yet another competency, information literacy, which falls under the umbrella of informatics. Depending on the objective—whether it is to feature current evidence on a single intervention (which uses systematic reviews) or teach the multifaceted approach to managing a disease (which uses clinical practice guidelines)—faculty model information literacy for students. Teaching how to access this information using open access also supports student learning as they increase their awareness of global nursing EBP and informatics issues. Because much scholarly information can now be accessed without charge for using this model, nurses worldwide can reach a higher level of information competency—a prime requirement for evidence-based practice (Nick, 2011). Information literacy aids faculty in wading through the sea of articles to find exactly what they need. Students also need this skill to use current evidence on which to base their practice.

PRACTICE SKILLED COMMUNICATION THAT REFLECTS AN AWARENESS OF SELF AND LEARNERS; COMMUNICATE EFFECTIVELY TO CONVEY IDEAS IN A VARIETY OF CONTEXTS

Competency in communication not only allows faculty to advance in their careers, it also serves as a role model for students. Students often learn or refine these skills while enrolled in nursing school. Continuously improving verbal expression when teaching, presenting at conferences, and speaking at university or department faculty meetings requires motivation, humility, and openness to change. Knowing how to electronically convey an idea efficiently, effectively, and without offense also takes skill. By demonstrating these skills, faculty will facilitate an environment of learning for students and colleagues.

Oral Communication

Most nursing schools enroll students from foreign countries. This creates the need for faculty to communicate with students from different linguistic and cultural backgrounds. A thick accent may make communicating effectively a challenge. If a faculty member or student receives consistent comments during peer or student evaluations about difficulty in understanding what he or she is saying, engaging in an accent modification program would show a willingness for accountability and continuous growth.

Accent reduction (or modification) programs are available for self-paced study. Carr and DeKemel-Ichikawa (2012) reported favorable results from an accent modification course for international nursing students. This strategy may be useful for foreign-born faculty or students.

Written Communication

To nurture writing skills in students, faculty must also model professional writing. By actively publishing, authors reap personal and professional rewards and impact the science of nursing by engaging in scholarship—a standard of practice for nurse educators (National League for Nursing, 2012). Conversely, the lack of publications may prevent faculty promotion, and knowing this makes faculty eager to be listed as the first or second author, potentially causing difficult situations when assumptions but no discussion occurs among coauthors. To increase responsible authorship, the International Committee of Medical Journal Editors published the "Vancouver Authorship" guidelines, which state that, to be considered for authorship, one needs to make substantial contribution to the conception and design, data collection, or analysis and interpretation of data (www.icmje.org/ethical_1author.html).

When writing academically or for professional publication, it is important to write with authority that is based on evidence (Fowler, 2010). Part of being collaborative is showing the willingness to review manuscripts for others and receive criticism from them for one's own manuscripts in return. Developing writing skills is like practicing an instrument. The more a faculty member practices writing, the more accurate, precise, and efficient he or she becomes at turning complex thoughts into a cohesive message.

MODEL REFLECTIVE THINKING PRACTICES, INCLUDING CRITICAL THINKING

Self-reflection, part of the critical thinking skill of self-regulation, is a vital component that encourages development of lifelong learning, successful change, and emotional intelligence. Self-regulation involves constant evaluation and self-monitoring of processes, responses, behaviors, intentions, and interpretations of events in daily life that encourage change and can serve as the backbone and structure for continued lifelong learning. Kuiper and Pesut (2004) referred to this process as metacognitive reflective reasoning skills and suggested the combination of cognitive skills and metacognitive reflective reasoning skills is the appropriate approach to teaching critical thinking and clinical reasoning skills. They assert that combining cognition and self-reflection provides the context for self-regulated learning theory, which is a strategy that can be learned, and using it in teaching can create a conducive learning environment for students (Allen, Ploeg, & Kaasalainen, 2012; Fernandez, Salamonson, & Griffiths, 2012).

Self-reflection allows faculty to understand their own belief systems, the assumptions that ground those beliefs, and how those assumptions and belief systems impact interactions with students. Assumptions and beliefs undergird all interactions with others, including colleagues, administrators, and students. Experienced as well as junior faculty must engage in self-reflection, as data suggest that as faculty advance in age, their ability to engage in self-evaluation diminishes, and they become more inflexible (Rossignol, 2006). The author attributes this behavior to environmental factors, such as increasingly heavy workloads, burnout, and stress. It may also reflect an outdated paradigm of teacher-centered comportment; faculty may believe they need to have all the answers rather than being colearners with their students (Schaefer & Zygmont, 2003).

A related but even more encompassing concept of self-reflection is emotional intelligence (EI). EI first appeared in the nursing literature in 1997 with a single article by Richardson and Borglatti. Since then nurse educators, clinicians, and managers have consistently studied and written about the concept. Vitello-Cicciu (2002) defined EI as the ability to perceive and regulate one's own emotions and others' in a way that positively influences communication, motivation, and teamwork. High EI offers many benefits: (a) reduced workplace stress, (b) decreased burnout, (c) improved clinical teaching effectiveness by faculty, (d) increased leadership effectiveness, and (e) improved physical and psychological well-being, social relationships, and employability (Allen et al., 2012; Fernandez et al., 2012; Foltin & Keller, 2012; Littlejohn, 2012; Nelis et al., 2011; Ziqiong, Changrong, & Chungping, 2012). When nurse educators include EI knowledge, skills, and attitudes in the curriculum, students learn how to act with discretion (Solbrekke & Sutphen, 2012). An added benefit for students is that developing EI has been shown to improve student academic and clinical performance (Beauvais, Brady, O'Shea, & Griffin, 2011). The take-away message from this body of research is that, to help students self-reflect and develop EI, faculty can and must also develop their own emotional intelligence (Nelis et al., 2011; Renaud, Rutledge, & Shepherd, 2012; Stoller, Taylor, & Farver, 2013).

In summary, self-reflection and EI are critical elements in the development of a nurse educator who wishes to demonstrate excellence in teaching. Reflection can alert the nurse educator to areas needing improvement. Haphazard or arbitrary approaches to the teaching–learning environment do not facilitate lifelong learning in either faculty or students.

Nurse educators speak of the need for teaching knowledge, skills, and attitudes (KSAs) of critical thinking (CT), but research shows it is not embedded tightly in nursing curricula. Rossignol (2006) found that most often, faculty posed questions to students that were lower-level cognition (facts) rather than asking for higher-level application, analysis, synthesis, and evaluation. Zygmont and Schaefer (2006) found few nurse faculty could provide examples of using CT in the classroom, nor could they clearly articulate a definition or the exact nature of CT KSAs. Other participants in this study spoke of CT as being synonymous with problem solving. Fortunately, most participants could provide examples of CT in the clinical area. These results are consistent within a larger university context of CT KSAs (Paul, Elder, & Bartell, 2013). Given these results, however, the question becomes: How can nurse educators include and improve modeling critical and reflective thinking to their students?

First, just like students, faculty must demonstrate a willingness, inclination, or predisposition for critical thinking. The literature calls this attitude "Disposition toward critical thinking." Three main areas of a disposition include (a) the willingness to question everything by being a truth-seeker, inquisitive, and open-minded, (b) the desire to give structure to thinking by being analytic and systematic, and (c) being confident yet judicious in the face of uncertainty (Facione & Gittens, 2013). If a nurse faculty is not disposed to thinking critically, he or she is unlikely to come to a well-justified conclusion when interpreting, analyzing, evaluating, using logic to infer inductively or deductively, explaining, or when trying to self-regulate. The good news is that CT dispositions can be taught to those interested in developing critical thinking skills (Vivien, Tham, Lau, Mei, & Kiat, 2010; Wagensteen, Johansson, Björkström, & Nordström, 2010). One of the ways nurse educators can model critical and reflective thinking is by being intentional about displaying the disposition and skill during faculty-to-faculty encounters (such as during councils and committee meetings). Once faculty are competent in using critical thinking, they can create those same opportunities for students in the learning environment.

CREATE OPPORTUNITIES FOR LEARNERS TO DEVELOP THEIR OWN CRITICAL THINKING SKILLS

Faculty can most impact a student's critical thinking skills by socializing them to the expectations in every course in the curriculum. The research by Rossignol

(2006) and Zygmont and Schaefer (2006) gives compelling evidence that nurse faculty do not speak of critical thinking in the classroom other than dangling the phrase "critical thinking" in front of students. And yet it is vitally important, as critical thinking forms the basis for clinical reasoning and clinical judgment (Rowles, 2012). If students do not have multiple opportunities for CT instruction, modeling, and practice, their clinical reasoning and judgment will be handicapped. Using CT terminology daily during the learning module, giving students the opportunity to practice interpreting data, graphs, and charts, analyzing diagnoses derived from deductive conclusions, and showing how nurses use induction to know what to assess when caring for a patient already diagnosed are exemplars. Creating self-reflection assignments, such as reflective journaling, is an excellent way for students to develop clinical judgment, as well as improve student–teacher communication (Lasater & Nielsen, 2009).

Measuring faculty competencies in facilitating reflection is now possible. Schaub-de Jong, Schönrock-Adema, Dekker, Verkerk, and Cohen-Schotanus (2011) developed a valid and reliable "Student perceptions of their Teachers' competencies to Encourage Reflective Learning in small Groups" (STERLinG) rating scale. The authors conducted the psychometric research using various health care professions (medical, dental, speech, and language professions). The structure of the tool comprises three areas: (a) faculty competency in supporting student self-insight, (b) creating a safe environment for reflection, and (c) encouraging student self-regulation. The authors conclude that the STERLinG rating scale is a practical tool that can be used to gather student perceptions of faculty competencies. Given the important nature of self-reflection and self-regulation in the larger context of critical thinking, nurse educators are encouraged to develop the use of critical thinking further and demonstrate competency, as there is now a tool that can be used to set potential benchmarks.

Another way to provide opportunities for critical thinking is for faculty and students to use the SEE-I method to gain clarity about an issue. Asking students to *state* it differently, *elaborate* on the topic, give an *example*, or *illustrate* it so the meaning can be visualized provides opportunities for increased understanding (Paul & Elder, 2013). Because research shows faculty tend to ask simple recall questions (Rossignol, 2006), framing higher-level questions is another way to support student learning. Finally, adding CT test items to examinations helps students make the connection between content involving critical thinking and clinical application.

Critical thinkers seek to gain all of the information and judge it for accuracy and validity before making a decision or judgment, which is also part of the process of gathering evidence. With evidence-based practice of nursing, Profetto-McGrath (2005) posits that critical thinking nurtures the EBP movement. EBP is a major paradigm shift for nursing education. By facilitating student willingness to ask difficult questions that answer root cause, risks, and benefits and coaching them to interpret, analyze, evaluate, and self-reflect, students will be able to practice based on current evidence, provide sound arguments, and develop confidence in their clinical decision-making.

CREATE A POSITIVE LEARNING ENVIRONMENT THAT FOSTERS A FREE EXCHANGE OF IDEAS

The next two sections deal with healthy and effective relationships: faculty-to-student and student-to-faculty; and faculty-to-faculty and faculty-to-clinical agency interactions. This section focuses on the importance of relationship building between faculty and student, using respect as the foundation regardless of existing power gradients. Respect is the cornerstone needed to create a safe environment for learning; if students do not feel safe while learning, they will avoid any interactions with the offending faculty when questions or issues arise (Altmiller, 2012; Clark & Springer, 2010). Surrounding students with respectful attitudes toward them, their peers, faculty, and their patients not only socializes them to future collegiality, but also enhances their learning. On the other hand, when students feel disrespected, their learning is hampered and they have difficulty attaining certain aspects of their professional role development (Altmiller, 2012; Clark & Springer, 2010; Del Prato, 2013). Hence, this topic merits full attention. What constitutes respectful and disrespectful behaviors by faculty, plus the effects of these behaviors on students, are reviewed.

Respectful Behaviors

Lerret and Frenn (2011) surveyed 27 doctoral students, purposefully chosen for their experience with numerous teachers and varying teaching styles during their baccalaureate, master's, and doctoral classes. Students wrote about teachers of excellence as those who know and honor students. Students listed behaviors that demonstrated faculty knew and honored students: listening, communicating value and respect to the student, and providing feedback in a way that encouraged rather than demeaned students. These characteristics set excellent teachers apart from the rest. The importance of respecting and valuing nursing students is paramount because these behaviors are some of the predictors for successful transition to becoming a nurse (Phillips, Esterman, Smith, & Kenny, 2013).

Disrespectful Behaviors

There is unfortunately more literature on disrespect and incivility than on characteristics of respectful faculty-to-student behavior. The task of the purposeful educator is to reflect on and translate information on disrespect into the concept of respect. None of the behaviors listed below, as reported by both educators and students, show respect toward students.

Clark and Springer (2010) queried 126 academic nurse leaders using a five-item survey regarding uncivil and disrespectful behaviors experienced in academia. Questions focused on perceived stressors of students and faculty and uncivil behaviors seen in students and faculty. Nurse administrators identifed three themes for faculty-to-student incivility. The largest types of behaviors reported included rudeness, avoidance behavior, belittling, demeaning, and being dismissive. Other less common behaviors included making unreasonable demands and not appreciating student contributions. The authors provided suggestions to address incivility and create a culture of mutual respect: providing student support, having strong leadership and role-modeling skills, and having intentional conversations and open forums. Del Prato (2013) reported these behaviors negatively impacted students' learning, self-esteem, self-efficacy, and confidence; these qualities all impact the concept of the professional self.

Altmiller (2012) interviewed 24 students, identifying nine themes of faculty-to-student incivility. Students recounted faculty not answering questions, making disparaging remarks, "putting down" students, talking negatively about students, targeting students, and scolding students in front of peers, staff, or patients. Also included in this list was the unequal treatment toward students (gender bias, racial discrimination, and favoritism). This behavior resulted in students losing respect for the faculty. Another theme identified in this research was the feeling of loss of control and disrespect when faculty yelled at students.

A disturbing finding in Altmiller's (2012) study was that students saw faculty behavior as a contributing cause to incivility in nursing education. In addition, the results brought attention to students' thinking—when they observed faculty incivility directed toward a student, students felt justified and experienced a sense of satisfaction in retaliating by behaving uncivilly toward the offending faculty.

Because demonstrating respect for students has far-reaching implications not only for students (learning, professional role development, and successful transition) but also for faculty (pleasant teaching environment), creating a culture of respect should be of prime concern. This can be done by (a) conducting formal training in how to establish respectful, connected relationships with students (Del Prato, 2013), (b) including the concept of respect in evaluations, and (c) engaging in personal self-reflection. If faculty feel disrespected by students and observe uncivil behaviors, self-reflection can help answer the question: Are students simply mirroring behaviors they are seeing in the faculty member?

This section underscores the impact respecting and valuing others for their unique contributions have on behavior. Faculty have an opportunity to model these attitudes and impact professional role formation. When students observe faculty modeling behaviors, whether negative or positive, students assume the behavior is acceptable. No wonder nurses in the clinical area continue to have relational problems among themselves and with other health care workers. Faculty must realize the gravity of role modeling and place importance on modeling respect. In response, students will incorporate this value into their professional role repertoire and treat faculty and future colleagues with respect.

SHOW ENTHUSIASM FOR TEACHING, LEARNING, AND THE NURSING PROFESSION THAT INSPIRES AND MOTIVATES STUDENTS

Enthusiasm is a prime characteristic needed to become an outstanding teacher. When no enthusiasm is shown for the material presented, how can students be motivated to struggle with and capture the true importance of the content? Enthusiasm, as a characteristic of excellence, has been validated by students and expert professors.

Lerret and Frenn (2011) queried 27 doctoral students in nursing using constant comparative content analysis. Enthusiasm was one of the four themes that emerged. Students in this study talked about a professor's ability to engage them in learning based on the professor's enthusiasm for the subject, which in turn motivated and inspired the students.

Another study also supported the need to be an enthusiastic educator. Johnson-Farmer and Frenn (2009) conducted grounded theory research to describe teaching excellence from the nurse educator's perspective. Seventeen teachers across the United States who had been identified by students as excellent teachers participated. Five themes identified the excellent educator. The fifth, dynamic engagement, spoke of the way nurse educators were perceived as real and alive, of showing true self.

We have already presented evidence in previous sections of this chapter on the impact engagement has on learning. Rossetti and Fox (2009) also studied nurse educator perspectives. In their study, they asked what made outstanding teachers.

Enthusiasm, passion, love, and joy of teaching were all words uncovered by these authors. So how can teachers display enthusiasm and passion? Displaying energy and excitement for the subject, varying tonal inflection, and having consistency between facial expressions and verbal messages demonstrate an enthusiasm and passion for the topic. When students see faculty passionate about the learning potential of each student, this inspires them to achieve more (Lerret & Frenn, 2011).

DEMONSTRATE PERSONAL ATTRIBUTES THAT FACILITATE LEARNING; FOSTER A SAFE LEARNING ENVIRONMENT

Personal attributes such as caring, confidence, patience, integrity, and flexibility are explicit values found in many vision and mission statements, and for good reason. They are qualities that facilitate students' ability to develop a trusting relationship with faculty, allowing faculty to demonstrate excellence in teaching. Caring is a universal nursing phenomenon and is reflected in faculty role modeling in the classroom, and in clinical and in laboratory settings (Sawatzky, Enns, Ashcroft, Davis, & Harder, 2009). In addition, these are all attributes students should demonstrate. When students witness faculty living these attributes, students receive the message "I am expected to live these attributes as well." What a powerful message that is. How can students respond to patients with a caring attitude if they do not identify those same behaviors in their faculty? Further, if students witness a faculty member's lack of confidence, or lack of integrity, this causes them to question the instruction and dismiss the faculty member as a professional. Outward signs of confidence make students believe in the teacher, and teachers must show they believe in their students. By doing this, students develop confidence in their own abilities (Houghton, Casey, Shaw, & Murphy, 2013). These behaviors contribute to a safe learning enviornnment. Because of the multiple roles of the current student population and the multiple demands placed by courses, flexibility in deadlines, participation, and choices in assignments have been identified as ways faculty can faciltate learning (Gaudine & Moralejo, 2011).

RESPOND EFFECTIVELY TO UNEXPECTED EVENTS THAT AFFECT INSTRUCTION

Flexibility is a required characteristic of nursing faculty in other ways as well. The unexpected can happen and has happened when schools experienced natural disasters and violence. Schools of nursing have adopted emergency plans to put into place if a weather-related event causes an unexpected, unplanned closure of the schools. Violence in schools also requires faculty to change educational plans in a quick fashion. Other unexpected events include a sudden illness or death of a faculty member. No matter what the event, faculty must always be prepared and able to respond effectively to unexpected events that affect instruction.

DEVELOP COLLEGIAL WORKING RELATIONSHIPS WITH CLINICAL AGENCY PERSONNEL TO PROMOTE POSITIVE LEARNING ENVIRONMENTS

Definitions of collegiality usually include phrases such as cooperative relationship of colleagues or cooperative interaction among colleagues. A colleague is an associate who belongs to a profession. In academia, collegiality is typically characterized by mutual respect, equality, and civility, in spite of having differences of opinion, while working to achieve a goal. According to the American Association of University Professors (AAUP, 1999), the last phrase is particularly important, as differences of opinion and diversity in thought form the basis for academic freedom. The AAUP agrees that the concept should include collaboration and constructive cooperation, but it clarifies that collegiality does not ensure homogeneity of thoughts, actions, or practices. Freedom of thought often creates conflict. Conflict might be avoided if faculty were to approach issues as nonemotional matters and discuss them realizing that all faculty are working toward a common goal but may have different opinions about how to achieve that goal (Jones, 1997).

Establishing Faculty-to-Faculty Collaborative Relationships

If respect, trust, and civility do not exist, then collaboration and collegiality cannot exist. Clark (2013b), whose work focuses principally in the area of nursing civility and incivility, has studied the building of civil environments from a faculty perspective and an academic leadership perspective (Clark & Springer, 2010). Investigating faculty perspectives on incivility, Clark (2013b) sent a combination quantitative and qualitative survey to academic nurse educators, with 588 faculty responding. The qualitative portion included questions such as: How do faculty describe uncivil faculty-to-faculty encounters, and what are the most effective ways to address this incivility? Results indicated faculty-to-faculty uncivil behaviors were similar though not exactly the same as faculty-to-student incivility. From this research, Clark showed civil environments must exist before collaborative relationships can occur. Faculty can create civility by (a) having direct, face-to-face communication during conflicts, (b) installing and sustaining effective, competent leadership, (c) measuring incivility in the workplace and creating policies to deal with it, (d) educating faculty and raising awareness, (e) transforming organizational culture, and (f) building and fostering faculty relationships and collaborations.

Academic leaders have a responsibility to create a culture of respect and civility, paving the way for a collegial environment. In Clark and Springer's (2010) earlier research, acting as participants, academic leaders suggested several interventions they as leaders could do to create and ensure a healthy, respectful work environment: (a) provide educational seminars and open forums, (b) model mutual respect, (c) hold faculty accountable for uncivil actions, (d) reward civility, (e) coach and mentor, and (f) create policy regarding uncivil behavior. Nursing departments having difficulty with incivility are encouraged to use the interventions identified by both educators and administrators to make the workplace collegial. Dealing with incivility takes courage, but confronting an uncivil coworker often puts an end to the problem (Clark, 2013b).

Continuing to live in an uncivil atmosphere at work is detrimental, as it can lead to low morale, high turnover, diminished quality of work, health issues, and isolation or alienation (Clark, 2013a). The importance of collegiality cannot be underscored too greatly, as the relational environment profoundly affects workplace satisfaction and retention (Duddle & Boughton, 2009). Because noncollegial relationships with leadership is one of the top three reasons faculty leave academia (Cropsey et al., 2008), the best practice is to take a healthy stance and deal with it.

A valid and reliable instrument has recently been developed to assess the workplace environment. In their psychometric study on the Nursing Workplace Relational Environment Scale, Duddle and Boughton (2009) identified four factors emerging from the exploratory factor analysis that explained the healthy workplace environment: (a) collegial behaviors, (b) relational atmosphere, (c) conflict resolution, and (d) resulting job satisfaction. These four factors accounted for almost 70 percent of the variance in the model. They go on to say that conflict in the workplace is inevitable, but how it is handled determines whether the outcomes are positive or negative. Because a paucity of nursing academic research exists on collegiality, a potential new body of research should be generated.

Establishing Collegial Relationships with Clinical Agencies

The shortage of clinical sites is evident; academic units continue to turn away thousands of qualified applicants each year (Kovner & Djukic, 2009). This means the academic nursing unit must develop creative ways to use clinical sites fully. Helping clinical agencies realize the mutually beneficial effects when partnerships are established is one way to nurture collegiality. To document best practices for developing increased partnerships with clinical sites, Teel, MacIntyre, Murray, and Rock (2011) probed schools and clinical sites regarding necessary elements to sustain healthy relationships. Their research provides the framework for interactions with clinical agencies: (a) establishing a mutually supportive relationship, (b) ensuring a good fit between the academic unit and the clinical agency, (c) having flexibility, and (d) establishing clear and open communication. Communication is foundational for any good working relationship and yet it cannot be stressed enough. These four themes can be turned into principles to complement traditional clinical site arrangements and to maintain healthy working relationships or implement with new models of academic–clinical partnerships (Maguire, Zambroski, & Cadena, 2012; Moore & Nahigian, 2013; Teel et al., 2011; Tuohy, 2011).

USE KNOWLEDGE OF EVIDENCE-BASED PRACTICE TO INSTRUCT LEARNERS

Rapid modifications in health care practice require the effective, efficient nurse educator to engage in change; this change is brought about by paradigm shifts in new content and teaching methods and includes such topics as technology and informatics, online education, evidence-based practice, and student-centered approaches to teaching. The responsible nurse educator advances these shifts by engaging in continuous learning of evidence-based nursing and teaching methods. Means to achieve currency include presenting at or attending conferences, keeping abreast of the literature, holding discussions with colleagues, and obtaining specialty certification.

When the focus is on student outcomes and what faculty can do to ensure student success, faculty are compelled to immerse themselves in the literature. In addition, because of rapid changes in health care with technology and informatics integrated in care delivery, students are expected to learn these systems and use them during their tenure as a student. Evidence-based practice and effective, efficient search skills help students obtain relevant and exponentially expanding clinical knowledge.

Health Informatics

In today's technology-rich clinical and educational environment, nurse educators must have a sufficient knowledge base of technology and informatics; the explosion of knowledge in these areas has changed the way health care professionals access, process, and use information (IOM, 2011, p. 191). In response, health informatics education has been identified as an essential component of nursing curricula (American Association of Colleges of Nursing, 2008; National League for Nursing Board of Governors, 2008). Two-thirds of nursing programs surveyed reported having some level of integration of technology in their program, while less than one-fourth had a stand-alone technology or informatics course (National League for Nursing Board of Governors, 2008). The TIGER initiative, in response to the call for education reform, provides resources and educational programs for faculty to use to incorporate technology in nursing care (www.thetigerinitiative. org/default.aspx). Programs such as the Health Information Technology Scholars program are available for faculty development. A recent integrative review regarding health informatics in nursing, conducted by De Gagne, Bisanar, Makowski, and Neumann (2011), concluded:

- There is a lack of consensus in the health literature regarding health informatics (HI) education for students and no recent research on the number of programs that include HI in their curriculum.
- There are positive and negative consequences when HI is included in nursing curricula, and special attention must be paid to ensuring safety of patient information. Because of the embedded safety aspects when using electronic health record (EHR) systems, faculty must offer training in areas of telehealth and EHR to provide optimal care to patients.
- Faculty need development of HI content as they have limited knowledge, skills, and motivation; partnering with clinical agencies for HI content will be crucial for the success of faculty and students achieving HI knowledge, skills, and attitudes.

Teaching of EBP

The topic of EBP was discussed earlier in the context of teaching practices being evidence based. This section briefly discusses the results of recent research on teaching EBP to students in the curriculum. Stichler, Fields, Kim, and Brown (2011) conducted descriptive exploratory research on two schools of nursing with baccalaureate and master's level nursing education. Forty nursing faculty (20 from each institution) volunteered to answer the EBP questionnaire, a 24-item instrument developed and validated by Upton and Upton (2006). Results showed faculty attitudes toward EBP were positive; however, they scored lower on EBP knowledge and skills when the aspect of fully implementing it in the curriculum was added. Because students need to apply EBP knowledge, skills, and attitudes in each clinical area, the sensible action would be to intentionally incorporate EBP activities in every course in the curriculum and offer faculty development workshops on EBP.

Maintaining Knowledge of Clinical or Educational Best Practices

Certification from a professional credentialing center is an indicator of specialized knowledge. The specialty certifications are based on evidence in the form of a practice analysis that is updated every few years.

To maintain the specialty certification requires evidence of lifelong learning in the form of continuing education units every three to five years and often includes practice hours. Maintaining specialty certification provides an incentive for faculty to stay current in their field of practice. Clinical certification programs have made a difference in nurse workplace empowerment (Krapohl, Manojlovich, Redman, & Zhang, 2010) and improved patient outcomes (Kendall-Gallagher & Blegen, 2009; Swanson & Tidwell, 2011; Zulkowski, Ayello, & Wexler, 2007).

Certification for nurse educators is similar in concept. The academic nurse educator certification program was begun in 2005 by the National League for Nursing. The competencies and certification exam are based on a practice analysis (Ortelli, 2006). To date, published studies testing the effect of academic nursing certification on student outcomes are sparse, yielding a fertile field for future research.

ACT AS A ROLE MODEL IN PRACTICE SETTINGS

Professional behavior, also termed *professional comportment,* is part of the learning process of becoming a professional nurse. It is a demonstration of desired behaviors, expressions, demeanor, verbalizations, and the way people conduct themselves in the course of their duties. Role modeling is the intentional observation of another's comportment because the observer seeks to mimic that behavior. It is an important teaching tool, as positive role modeling inspires greatness in others through the role model's passion and engagement in serving.

It is important to note that role modeling is always present. Faculty are constantly observed by students, and students hold faculty accountable, often to a higher level. At any given time, students can be observing a teacher's dialogue with a patient, nurse, or another colleague; watching an instructor complete a procedure; or noting nonverbal behavior (Gardner & Suplee, 2010); they then assign behaviors as either positive or negative. If a student observes a negative interaction by a third party, faculty can seize the opportunity to guide the student to identify more acceptable behavior.

Based on a concept analysis, Clickner and Shirey (2013) identified positive role-modeling attributes: (a) demonstration of mutual respect, (b) beliefs and actions that are harmonious and consistent, (c) marked commitment, and (d) evidence of a spirit of collaboration. These authors advanced the argument that professional comportment is a dimension of nursing practice that is of equal importance as competently performing technical tasks. Faculty have many opportunities to verbally instruct students about professional comportment: during course orientation, individual classes or modules, at department-sponsored colloquia, and in the clinical setting. But when students use faculty as the "referent group," faculty are afforded opportunities to demonstrate professional nursing comportment. A powerful learning experience occurs even when faculty are unaware learning is taking place (Gardner & Suplee, 2010). And when faculty internalize the power of role modeling, they comport themselves by displaying caring and respectful words, positive communication, and professional attire; creating effective relationships with patients and colleagues; displaying self-regulation; and learning accountability (Clickner & Shirey, 2013).

In addition, role modeling is not only effective for professional comportment, but also for (a) helping students develop positive attitudes toward EBP (Winters & Echeverri, 2012) and (b) building trust and willingness, which is the basis for the transformation into a learning environment (Schoonbeek & Henderson, 2011), developing integrity and academic honesty (Woith, Jenkins, & Kerber, 2012), and determining professional values (Duquette, 2004).

SUMMARY

This chapter focused on the current research in areas that support the nurse educator. Learners learn best when they participate in a variety of learning experiences, using their natural disposition for learning. Faculty are encouraged to move away from conveying an ever-growing body of content (teacher-inspired environment) and to move toward teaching concepts and applications and helping students learn how to find the information and give it meaning. A variety of contexts support learning, no one is superior to another. To use teaching methods steeped in evidence, faculty have the dual responsibility of monitoring both clinical and educational literature to remain current and of paying attention to other databases that feature pedagogical research, an important strategy on which nurse educators can ground their teaching and innovate based on evidence. Engaging students in the learning rather than having them passively listen to a lecture provides the framework for collaboration, teamwork, communication, and critical thinking. By eliminating bias from the educational environment, faculty establish a milieu where ethnically and racially diverse students, both genders, and differing age groups can thrive.

Incorporating technology into the active learning environment supports student engagement, lifelong learning, and information literacy skills, which are all needed to accomplish evidence-based nursing practice. Students often struggle with written assignments, but faculty can use this opportunity to model standard professional behavior by being engaged in publishing and demonstrating how writing can impact the science of nursing.

Practice Test Questions

1. Which student role has been shown to be least effective for students while practicing nursing in a clinical simulation environment?
   A. Documentation nurse role
   B. Family member role
   C. Patient role
   D. Observer role

2. What curricular change in promoting education reform would best prepare students for a complex health care environment, support critical thinking, and encourage lifelong learning?
   A. Increase community clinical experiences
   B. Include a health informatics technology course
   C. Develop learning experiences that build upon previously learned experiences
   D. Provide classroom experiences that provide faculty–student interaction

3. The nursing instructor expects the students in a pathophysiology course to be able to correlate the physiological changes experienced by complex medical patients with their clinical manifestations and complications. Which strategy should the instructor choose to best foster critical thinking?
   A. Help students use inductive thinking to determine what to assess
   B. Lecture about expected findings for each diagnostic test
   C. Call for students to write a 1-minute paper
   D. Show a short 20-minute movie about a pertinent clinical case

4. A nurse educator is attempting to help students learn to appreciate and value team member differences and increase team functioning. What is an evidence-based strategy that will facilitate this endeavor?
   A. Incorporate technology in the learning session to help students find current information
   B. Provide classroom activities that encourage faculty–student interaction
   C. Assign group classroom activities for which each group comprises students with different learning styles
   D. Communicate to students that completion of classroom activities will provide the necessary tools for success

5. The evidence shows one of the ways excellent teachers stand apart from other teachers is by the way they interact with students. Which statement by a teacher provides an example of excellence?
   A. Given your grade on the midterm exam, I think it would be in your best interest to drop this course and return the following term.
   B. Your technique for this skill was solid and you show concern for safety, which is paramount. I know with practice, you will become proficient very quickly.
   C. Can you find a classmate who can help you understand this material? Maybe explanation from a different person will help because I haven't been successful at explaining it clearly.
   D. I would like to see you become more involved in the actual care for your patients. Whenever I come to this unit, I see you looking over the chart rather than being in the patient's room.

(continued on page 26)

6. Which question by the clinical instructor would allow the student to demonstrate critical thinking and development of clinical judgment?
   A. Do you think this patient needs the stool softener prescribed for him?
   B. What teaching does this patient need so that her blood sugar can be more stable?
   C. What would be the best way to manage pain symptoms for this patient following the transurethral resection of the prostate?
   D. How have priorities changed for this patient from yesterday to today now that he is one day postoperative?

7. The nurse educator is concerned that students are not paying attention in class during the lecture; they visit Internet websites, text on their cell phones, stare at the desk with glazed eyes, or look bored. What strategy could the nurse educator use to engage the students and help them practice decision making?
   A. Give the PowerPoint more action and photos
   B. Use Socratic questioning with the students
   C. Call for a surprise quiz on the material covered in class
   D. Use a personal response system with NCLEX-style questions

8. An academic nurse administrator is reviewing student evaluations of four faculty. Which written comments by students would reassure the administrator of the faculty's expertise in motivating students to learn?
   A. The teacher is very enthusiastic in interactions with us as students. It makes me want to show the same enthusiasm to my studies.
   B. The teacher is kind and gentle and also comes well prepared to class and uses technology appropriately.
   C. The teacher is prompt about answering my questions by email or texting. He is also very knowledgeable about the content.
   D. The teacher has extensive information on the PowerPoint slides, which helps me concentrate on class instead of taking notes.

9. A faculty member notices this year's class of students is disruptive, coming in late and leaving early, is unprepared, and uses their cell phones or computers for activities unrelated to listening to the lecture. What would be an appropriate response by the faculty to remedy the situation?
   A. Stop the lecture and politely ask students to pay attention, then start again
   B. Continue the lecture and ignore the behaviors, because it is not disturbing other students
   C. Involve the students by asking them to use their cell phones to look up information
   D. Review organizational values with the students and remind them of their professional responsibility

10. A nurse educator is at a faculty meeting, and there is heated discussion about how to include informatics in the curriculum. What would be the most collegial response by the faculty member during the discussion?
   A. Cooperate with whatever the decision is, as usually the group decision is the correct decision
   B. Depersonalize the decision and focus on the goal and the many ways to achieve it
   C. When there is a break in the discussion, start talking and say, "Well I think we should…"
   D. Side talk with a colleague and state how you think informatics should be incorporated

References

Allen, D. E., Ploeg, J., & Kaasalainen, S. (2012). The relationship between emotional intelligence and clinical teaching effectiveness in nursing faculty. *Journal of Professional Nursing, 28*(4), 231–240.

Altmiller, G. (2012). Student perceptions of incivility in nursing education: Implications for educators. *Nursing Education Perspectives, 33*(1), 15–20. doi:10.5480/1536-5026-33.1.15

Amaro, D., Abriam-Yago, K., & Yoder, M. (2006). Perceived barriers for ethnically diverse students in nursing programs. *Journal of Nursing Education, 45*(7), 247–254.

American Association of Colleges of Nursing. (2008). Essentials of baccalaureate education for professional practice. Retrieved from http://www.aacn.nche.edu/education-resources/BaccEssentials08.pdf

American Association of Colleges of Nursing. (2009). Annual report advancing higher education in nursing. Retrieved from http://www.aacn.nche.edu/Media/Annualreport.htm

American Association of University Professors. (1999). On collegiality as a criterion for faculty evaluation. Retrieved from http://www.aaup.org/report/collegiality-criterion-faculty-evaluation

Andersen, E. A., Strumpel, C., Fensom, I., & Andrews, W. (2011). Implementing team based learning in large classes: Nurse educators' experiences. *International Journal of Nursing Education Scholarship, 8*(1), art. 28. doi:10.2202/1548-923X.2197

Baker, C. M., McDaniel, A. M., Pesut, D. J., & Fisher, M. L. (2007). Learning skills profiles of master's students in nursing administration: Assessing the impact of problem-based learning. *Nursing Education Perspectives, 28*(4), 190–195.

Beauvais, A. M., Brady, N., O'Shea, E. R., & Griffin, M. T. (2011). Emotional intelligence and nursing performance among nursing students. *Nurse Education Today, 31*(4), 396–401. doi:10.1016/j.nedt.2010.07.013

Beischel, K. (2013). Variables affecting learning in a simulation experience: A mixed methods study. *Western Journal of Nursing Research, 35*(2), 226–247. doi:10.1177/0193945911408444

Benner, P., Sutphen, P., Leonard, V., & Day, L. (2010). *Educating nurses: A call for radical transformation.* San Francisco, CA: Jossey-Bass.

Billings, D. M. (2012). Developing learner-centered courses. In D. M. Billings & J. A. Halstead (Eds.), *Teaching in nursing: A guide for faculty* (pp. 160–169). St. Louis, MO: Elsevier.

Bloom, B. S., Engelhart, M. B., Furst, E. J., Hill, W. H., & Krathwohl, D. R. (1956). *Taxonomy of educational objectives: The classification of educational goals. Handbook I: Cognitive domain.* New York: David McKay.

Bosher, S. D. (2009). Removing language as a barrier to success on multiple-choice nursing exams. In S. D. Bosher & M. D. Pharris (Eds.), *Transforming nursing education: The culturally inclusive environment* (pp. 264-266). New York, NY: Springer.

Bosher, S., & Bowles, M. (2008). The effects of linguistic modification on ESL students' comprehension of nursing course test items. *Nursing Education Perspectives, 29*(3), 165–172.

Burruss, N., & Popkess, A. (2012). The diverse learning needs of students. In D. M. Billings & J. A. Halstead (Eds.), *Teaching in nursing: A guide for faculty* (4th ed., pp. 15-33). St. Louis, MO: Elsevier.

Candela, L. (2012). From teaching to learning: Theoretical foundations. In D. M. Billings & J. A. Halstead (Eds.), *Teaching in nursing: A guide for faculty* (4th ed., pp. 202-243). St. Louis, MO: Elsevier.

Carr, S. M., & DeKemel-Ichikawa, K. (2012). Improving communication through accent modification: Growing the nursing workforce. *Journal of Cultural Diversity, 19*(3), 79–84.

Centrella-Nigro, A. M. (2012). Collaborative testing as posttest review. *Nursing Education Perspectives, 33*(5), 340–341.

Clark, C. M. (2013a). *Creating and sustaining civility in nursing edcuation.* Indianapolis, IN: Sigma Theta Tau International.

Clark, C. M. (2013b). National study on faculty-to-faculty incivility: Strategies to foster collegiality and civility. *Nurse Educator, 38*(3), 98–102. doi:10.1097/NNE.0b013e31828dc1b2

Clark, C. M., & Springer, P. J. (2010). Academic nurse leaders' role in fostering a culture of civility in nursing education. *Journal of Nursing Education, 49*(6), 319–325. doi:10.3928/01484834-20100224-01

Clickner, D. A., & Shirey, M. A. (2013). Professional comportment: The missing element in nursing practice. *Nursing Forum, 48*(2), 106–113. Retrieved from http://dx.doi.org/10.1111/nuf.12014

Collier, J. (2010). Wiki technology in the classroom: Building collaboration skills. *Journal of Nursing Education, 49*(12), 718.

Cools, E., Evans, C., & Redmond, J. (2009). Using styles for more effective learning in multicultural and e-learning environments. *Multicultural Education & Technology Journal, 3*(1), 5–16.

Cropsey, K. L., Masho, S. W., Shiang, R., Sikka, V., Kornstein, S. G., & Hampton, C. L. (2008). Why do faculty leave? Reasons for attrition of women and minority faculty from a medical school: Four-year results. *Journal of Women's Health, 17*(7), 1111–1118.

Dalley, K., Candela, L., & Benzel-Lindley, J. (2008). Learning to let go: The challenge of de-crowding the curriculum. *Nurse Education Today, 28*(1), 62–69.

De Gagne, J. C., Bisanar, W. A., Makowski, J. T., & Neumann, J. L. (2011). Integrating informatics into the BSN curriculum: A review of the literature. *Nurse Education Today, 32*, 675–682. doi:10.1016/j.nedt.2011.09.003

DeBourgh, G. A. (2008). Use of classroom "clickers" to promote acquisition of advanced reasoning skills. *Nurse Education in Practice, 8*, 76–87.

Del Prato, D. (2013). Students' voices: The lived experience of faculty incivility as a barrier to professional formation in associate degree nursing education. *Nurse Education Today, 33*(3), 286–290. doi:10.1016/j.nedt.2012.05.030

Dobbins, W. N., Souder, E., & Smith, R. M. (2005). Living with fair use and TEACH: A quest for compliance. *CIN: Computers, Informatics, Nursing, 23*(3), 120–124.

Duddle, M., & Boughton, M. (2009). Development and psychometric testing of the Nursing Workplace

Relational Environment Scale (NWRES). *Journal of Clinical Nursing, 18*(6), 902–909. doi:10.1111/j.1365-2702.2008.02368.x

DuHamel, M. B., Hirnle, C., Karvonen, C., Sayre, C., Wyant, S., Smith, N. C.,…Whitney, J. (2011). Enhancing medical-surgical nursing practice: Using practice tests and clinical examples to promote active learning and program evaluation. *Journal of Continuing Education in Nursing, 42*(10), 457–462. doi:10.3928/00220124-20110701-01

Duquette, L. M. (2004). *Effects of nursing education on the formation of professional values.* Unpublished doctoral dissertation, University of Toronto, Ontario, Canada.

Efstathiou, N., & Bailey, C. (2012). Promoting active learning using Audience Response System in large bioscience classes. *Nurse Education Today, 32*(1), 91–95. doi:10.1016/j.nedt.2011.01.017

Facione, P., & Gittens, C. (2013). *Think critically.* Upper Saddle River, NJ: Prentice-Hall.

Ferguson, L., & Day, R. A. (2005). Evidence-based nursing education: Myth or reality? *Journal of Nursing Education, 44*(3), 107–115.

Fernandez, R., Salamonson, Y., & Griffiths, R. (2012). Emotional intelligence as a predictor of academic performance in first-year accelerated graduate entry nursing students. *Journal of Clinical Nursing, 21,* 3485–3492. doi:10.1111/j.1365-2702.2012.04199.x

Foltin, A., & Keller, R. (2012). Leading change with emotional intelligence. *Nursing Management, 43*(11), 20–25. doi:10.1097/01.NUMA.0000421675.33594.63

Fowler, J. (2010). Writing for professional publication. Part 4: Supporting your statements. *British Journal of Nursing, 19*(21), 1374.

Gallagher-Lepak, S., Reilly, J., & Killion, C. M. (2009). Nursing student perceptions of community in online learning. *Contemporary Nurse, 32*(1–2), 133–146. Retrieved from http://dx.doi.org/10.5172/conu.32.1-2.133

Gardner, M. R., & Suplee, P. D. (2010). *Handbook of clinical teaching in nursing and health sciences.* Boston, MA: Jones and Bartlett.

Gaudine, A. P., & Moralejo, D. G. (2011). What can faculty members and programs do to improve students' learning? *ISRN Nursing, 2011,* 2011, 649431. doi:10.5402/2011/649431

Gibson, S. E. (2009). Enhancing intergenerational communication in the classroom: Recommendations for successful teacher-student relationships. *Nursing Education Perspectives, 30*(1), 37–39.

Giddens, J., & Brady, D. (2007). Rescuing nursing education from content saturation: A case for a concept-based curriculum. *Journal of Nursing Education, 46*(2), 65–69.

Giddens, J., Brady, D., Brown, P., Wright, M., Smith, D., & Harris, J. (2008). A new curriculum for a new era of nursing education. *Nursing Education Perspectives, 29*(4), 200–204.

Godwin-Jones, R. (2005). Messaging, gaming, peer-to-peer sharing: Language learning strategies and tools for the millennial generation. *Language, Learning and Technology, 9*(1), 17–22.

Gruendemann, B. J. (2011). Nursing student experiences with face-to-face learning. *Journal of Nursing Education, 50*(12), 676–680. doi:10.3928/01484834-20110930-02

Halstead, J. A., Phillips, J. M., Koller, A., Hardin, K., Porter, M. L., & Dwyer, J. S. (2011). Preparing nurse educators to use simulation technology: A consortium model for practice and education. *Journal of Continuing Education in Nursing, 42*(11), 496–502. Retrieved from http://dx.doi.org/10.3928/00220124-20110502-01

Hayden, J. (2010). Use of simulation in nursing education: National survey results. *Journal of Nursing Regulation, 1*(3), 52–57.

Health Resources and Service Administration (HRSA). (2010). *The registered nurse population: Findings from the National Sample Survey of registered nurses.* Rockville, MD: Author.

Houghton, C. E., Casey, D., Shaw, D., & Murphy, K. (2013). Students' experiences of implementing clinical skills in the real world of practice. *Journal of Clinical Nursing, 22*(13-14), 1961–1969. doi:10.1111/jocn.12014

Institute of Medicine (IOM). (2011). *The future of nursing: Leading change, advancing health.* Washington, DC: National Academies Press.

Ironside, P. A. (2004). "Covering Content" and teaching thinking: Deconstructing the additive curriculum. *Journal of Nursing Education, 43*(1), 5–12.

Johnson-Farmer, B., & Frenn, M. (2009). Teaching excellence: What great teachers teach us. *Journal of Professional Nursing, 25,* 267–272. doi:10.1016/j.profnurs.2009.01.020

Jones, D. A. (1997). Plays well with others, or the importance of collegiality within a reference unit. *Reference Librarian, 28*(59), 163–175. doi:10.1300/J120v28n59_18

Jones, S., Henderson, D., & Sealover, P. (2009). "Clickers" in the classroom. *Teaching and Learning in Nursing, 4,* 2–5.

Kardong-Edgren, S. E., Oermann, M. H., Tennant, M. N., Snelson, C., Hallmark, E., Rogers, N., & Hurd, D. (2009). Using a wiki in nursing education and research. *International Journal of Nursing Education Scholarship, 6*(1), 1–10. doi:10.2202/1548-923X.1787

Kendall-Gallagher, D., & Blegen, M. A. (2009). Competence and certification of registered nurses and safety of patients in intensive care units. *American Journal of Critical Care, 18*(2), 106–113. doi:10.4037/ajcc2009487

Knowles, M. S. (1980). *The modern practice of adult education.* Chicago, IL: Follett.

Kovner, C., & Djukic, M. (2009). The nursing career process from application through the first 2 years of employment. *Journal of Professional Nursing, 25*(4), 197–203. doi:10.1016/j.profnurs.2009.05.002

Krapohl, G., Manojlovich, M., Redman, R., & Zhang, L. (2010). Nursing specialty certification and nursing-sensitive patient outcomes in the intensive care unit. *American Journal of Critical Care, 19*(6), 490–494. Retrieved from http://dx.doi.org/10.4037/ajcc2010406

Kuiper, R. A., & Pesut, D. J. (2004). Promoting cognitive and metacognitive reflective reasoning skills in nursing practice: Self-regulated learning theory. *Journal of Advanced Nursing, 45*(4), 381–391. doi:10.1046/j.1365-2648.2003.02921.x

Kyprianidou, M., Demetriadis, S., Tsiatsos, T., & Pombortsis, A. (2012). Group formation based on learning styles: Can it improve students' teamwork? *Educational Technology Research & Development, 60*(1), 83–110. doi:10.1007/s11423-011-9215-4

LaCharity, L. A., Kumagai, C. K., & Bartz, B. (2013). *Prioritization, delegation, and assignment: Practice exercises for the NCLEX examination* (3rd ed.). St. Louis, MO: Elsevier.

Lake, S., Moss, C., & Duke, J. (2009). Nursing prioritization of the patient need for care: A tacit knowledge embedded in the clinical decision-making literature. *International Journal of Nursing Practice, 15*(5), 376–388.

Lampe, S., & Tsaouse, B. (2010). Linguistic bias in multiple-choice test questions. *Creative Nursing, 16*(2), 63–67. Retrieved from http://dx.doi.org/10.1891/1078-4535.16.2.63

Lancaster, J. W., Wong, A., & Roberts, S. (2012). "Tech" versus "talk": A comparison study of two different lecture styles within a master of science nurse practicitioner course. *Nurse Education Today, 32*(5), e14-e18. doi:10.1016/j.nedt.2011.09.018

Lasater, K., & Nielsen, A. (2009). Reflective journaling for clinical judgment development and evaluation. *Journal of Nursing Education, 48*(1), 40–44.

Lerret, S. M., & Frenn, M. (2011). Challenge with care: Reflections on teaching excellence. *Journal of Professional Nursing, 27*(6), 378–384. doi:10.1016/j.profnurs.2011.04.014

Levitt, C., & Adelman, D. S. (2010). Role-playing in nursing theory: Engaging online students. *Journal of Nursing Education, 49*(4), 229–232. Retrieved from http://dx.doi.org/10.3928/01484834-20091217-03

Lewallen, L. P., & DeBrew, J. K. (2012). Successful and unsuccessful clinical nursing students. *Journal of Nursing Education, 51*(7), 389–395. doi:10.3928/01484834-20120427-01

Littlejohn, P. (2012). The missing link: Using emotional intelligence to reduce workplace stress and workplace violence in our nursing and other health care profesesions. *Journal of Professional Nursing, 28*(6), 360–368. doi:10.1016/j.profnurs.2012.04.006

Lubeck, P., Tschetter, L., & Mennenga, H. (2013). Team-based learning: An innovative approach to teaching maternal-newborn nursing care. *Journal of Nursing Education, 52*(2), 112–115. doi:10.3928/01484834-20130121-02

Lujan, J. (2008). Linguistic and cultural adaptation needs of Mexican American nursing students related to multiple-choice tests. *Journal of Nursing Education, 47*(7), 327–330.

Lyons, M. G. (2010). Open access is almost here: Navigating through copyright, fair use, and the TEACH Act. *Journal of Continuing Education in Nursing, 41*(2), 57–64. doi:10.3928/00220124-20100126-03

Maguire, D. J., Zambroski, C. H., & Cadena, S. V. (2012). Using a clinical collaborative model for nursing education: Application for clinical teaching. *Nurse Educator, 37*(2), 80–85. doi:10.1097/NNE.0b013e3183461bb6

Mareno, N., Bremner, M., & Emerson, C. (2010). The use of audience response systems in nursing education: Best practice guidelines. *International Journal of Nursing Education Scholarship, 7*(1), art. 32. Retrieved from http://dx.doi.org/10.2202/1548-923X.2049

McLaughlin, K., Muldoon, O. T., & Moutray, M. (2010). Gender, gender roles and completion of nursing education: A longitudinal study. *Nurse Education Today, 30*, 303–307. doi:10.1016/j.nedt.2009.08.005

Meadus, R. J., & Twomey, J. C. (2011). Men student nurses: The nursing education experience. *Nursing Forum, 46*(4), 269–279. Retrieved from http://dx.doi.org/10.1111/j.1744-6198.2011.00239.x

Moore, J., & Nahigian, E. (2013). Nursing student perceptions of nurse-to-nurse collaboration in dedicated education units and in traditional clinical instruction units. *Journal of Nursing Education, 52*(6), 346–350. doi:10.3928/01484834-20130509-01

Mulready-Shick, J., Kafel, K. W., & Banister, G. (2009). Enhancing quality and safety competency development at the unit level: An initial evaluation of student learning and clinical teaching on dedicated education units. *Journal of Nursing Education, 48*(12), 716–719. doi10.3928/01484834-20091113-11

National Council of State Boards of Nursing. (2012). *NCLEX-RN® Examination: Test plan for the National Council Licensure Examination for Registered Nurses.* Chicago, IL: Author.

National League for Nursing. (2006). *Excellence in nursing education model.* New York: Author.

National League for Nursing. (2012). *The scope of practice for academic nurse educators.* Philadelphia, PA: Lippincott Williams & Wilkins.

National League for Nursing Board of Governors. (2008). *Preparing the next generation of nurses to practice in a technology-rich environment: An informatics agenda* [Position Statement]. Retrieved from http://www.nln.org/aboutnln/PositionStatements/informatics_052808.pdf

Nelis, D., Kotsou, I., Quoidbach, J., Hansenne, M., Weytens, F., Dupuis, P., & Mikolajczak, M. (2011). Increasing emotional competence improves psychological and physical well-being, social relationships, and employability. *Emotion, 11*(2), 354–366.

Nick, J. M. (2011, November 23). Open access part I: The movement, the issues, and the benefits. *Online Journal of Issues in Nursing, 17*(1), 8. doi:10.3912/OJIN.Vol17No01PPT02

Ortelli, T. A. (2006). Defining the professional responsibilities of academic nurse educators: The results of a national practice analysis. *Nursing Education Perspectives, 27*(5), 242–246.

Özbıçakçı, S., Bilik, Ö., & İntepeler, S. S. (2012). Assessment of goals in problem-based learning. *Nurse Education Today, 32*, 79–82. doi:10.1016/j.nedt.2012.03.017

Patterson, B. J., & Klein, J. M. (2012). Evidence for teaching: What are faculty using? *Nursing Education Perspectives, 33*(4), 240–245.

Paul, R., & Elder, L. (2013). The standards for thinking. In R. Paul & L. Elder (Eds.), *Critical thinking: Tools for taking charge of your professional and personal life* (2nd ed., pp. 98-129). Upper Saddle River, NJ: Pearson Prentice-Hall.

Paul, R., Elder, L., & Bartell, T. (2013, June 6). Study of 38 public universities and 28 private universities to determine faculty emphasis on critical thinking in instruction. Retrieved from http://www.criticalthinking.org/pages/study-of-38-public-universities-and-28-private-universities-to-determine-faculty-emphasis-on-critical-thinking-in-instruction/598

Pennington, T., & Spurlock, D. (2010). A systematic review of the effectiveness of remediation interventions to improve NCLEX-RN pass rates. *Journal of Nursing Education, 49*(9), 485–492. doi:10.3928/01484834-20100630-05

Phillips, C., Esterman, A., Smith, C., & Kenny, A. (2013). Predictors of successful transition to registered nurse. *Journal of Advanced Nursing, 69*(6), 1314–1322. doi:10.1365-2648.2012.06123.x

Popkess, A. M., & McDaniel, A. (2011). Are nursing students engaged in learning? A secondary analysis of data from the National Survey of Student Engagement. *Nursing Education Perspectives, 32*(2), 89–94. Retrieved from http://dx.doi.org/10.5480/1536-5026-32.2.89

Profetto-McGrath, J. (2005). Critical thinking and evidence-based practice. *Journal of Professional Nursing, 21*(6), 364–371.

Pryjmachuk, S., Easton, K., & Littlewood, A. (2009). Nurse education: Factors associated with attrition. *Journal of Advanced Nursing, 65*(1), 149–160. doi:10.1111/j.1365-2648.2008.04852.x

Ramsden, P. (2013). *Learning to teach in higher education* (3rd ed.) London: Routledge.

Reilly, J. R., Gallagher-Lepak, S., & Killion, C. (2012). "Me and my computer": Emotional factors in online learning. *Nursing Education Perspectives, 33*(2), 100–105. Retrieved from http://dx.doi.org/10.5480/1536-5026-33.2.100

Renaud, M. T., Rutledge, C., & Shepherd, L. (2012). Preparing emotionally intelligent doctor of nursing practice leaders. *Journal of Nursing Education, 51*(8), 454–460. Retrieved from http://dx.doi.org/10.3928/01484834-20120523-03

Revell, S. M., & McCurry, M. K. (2010). Engaging millennial learners: Effectiveness of personal response system technology with nursing students in small and large classrooms. *Journal of Nursing Education, 49*(5), 272–275. Retrieved from http://dx.doi.org/10.3928/01484834-20091217-07

Richardson, H., Gilmartin, M., & Fulmer, T. (2012). Shifting the clinical teaching paradigm in undergraduate nursing education to address the nursing faculty shortage. *Journal of Nursing Education, 51*(4), 226–231.

Richardson, K. L., & Borglatti, J. C. (1997). Emotional Intelligence in the workplace. *Nursing Spectrum, New England Edition, 1*(7), 16.

Roberts, D. S., Ingram, R. R., Flack, S. A., & Hayes, R. J. (2013). Implementation of mastery learning in nursing education. *Journal of Nursing Education, 52*(4), 234–237. doi:10.3928/01484834-20130319-02

Rossetti, J., & Fox, P. G. (2009). Factors related to successful teaching by outstanding professors: An interpretive study. *Journal of Nursing Education, 48*(1), 11–16.

Rossignol, M. (2006). Verbal and cognitive activities between and among students and faculty in clinical conferences. *Journal of Nursing Education, 39*(6), 245–250.

Rowles, C. J. (2012). Strategies to promote critical thinking and active learning. In D. M. Billings & J. A. Halstead, *Teaching in nursing: A guide for faculty* (4th ed., pp. 258-284). St. Louis, MO: Elsevier.

Rundle, S., & Dunn, R. (2008). *Building excellence (BE)® BE 2000 research manual 1996-2008.* Rochester, NY: Performance Concepts International.

Sandahl, S. S. (2010). Collaborative testing as a learning strategy in nursing education. *Nursing Education Perspectives, 31*(3), 142–147.

Sawatzky, J. V., Enns, C. L., Ashcroft, T. J., Davis, P. L., & Harder, B. N. (2009). Teaching excellence in nursing education: A caring framework. *Journal of Professional Nursing, 25*(5), 260–266. doi:10.1016/j.profnurs.2009.01.017

Schaefer, K. M., & Zygmont, D. M. (2003). Analyzing the teaching style of nursing faculty: Does it promote a student-centered or teacher-centered learning environment? *Nursing Education Perspectives, 24*(5), 238–245.

Schaub-de Jong, M. A., Schönrock-Adema, J., Dekker, H., Verkerk, M., & Cohen-Schotanus, J. (2011). Development of a student rating scale to evaluate teachers' competencies for facilitating reflective learning. *Medical Education, 45*(2), 155–165. doi:10.1111/j.1365-29232010.03774.x

Schoonbeek, S., & Henderson, A. (2011). Shifting workplace behavior to inspire learning: A journey to building a learning culture. *Journal of Continuing Education in Nursing, 42*(1), 43–48. Retrieved from http://dx.doi.org/10.3928/00220124-20101001-02

Seiler, K., & Billings, D. M. (2004). Student experiences in web-based nursing courses: Benchmarking best practices. *International Journal of Nursing Education Scholarship, 1*(1), art. 20.

Sisk, R. J. (2011). Team-based learning: Systematic research review. *Journal of Nursing Education, 50*(12), 665–669. doi:10.3928/01484834-20111017-01

Skiba, D. L. (2007). Nursing education 2.0: Second life. *Nursing Education Perspectives, 28*(3), 156–157.

Solbrekke, T. D., & Sutphen, M. (2012). Learning in a web of commitments. *Journal of Nursing Education, 51*(4), 185–189. doi:10.3928/01484834-20120210-01

Stichler, J. F., Fields, W., Kim, S. C., & Brown, C. E. (2011). Faculty knowledge, attitudes, and perceived barriers to teaching evidence-based nursing. *Journal of Professional Nursing, 27*(2), 92–100. doi:10.1016/j.profnur.2010.09.02

Stoller, J. K., Taylor, C. A., & Farver, C. F. (2013). Emotional intelligence competencies provide a developmental curriculum for medical training. *Medical Teacher, 35*(3), 243–247. Retrieved from http://dx.doi.org/10.3109/0142159X.2012.737964

Swanson, J. W., & Tidwell, C. A. (2011, September 30). Improving the culture of patient safety through the Magnet journey. *Online Journal of Issues in Nursing, 16*(3), 1. doi:10.3912/OJIN.Vol16No03Man01

Tanicala, M. L., Scheffer, B. K., & Roberts, M. S. (2011). PASS/FAIL nursing student clinical behaviors Phase I: Moving toward a culture of safety. *Nursing*

Education Research, 32(3), 155–161. Retrieved from http://dx.doi.org/10.5480/1536-5026-32.3.155

Tanner, C. A. (2004). The meaning of curriculum: Content to be covered or stories to be heard? *Journal of Nursing Education, 43*(1), 3–4.

Teel, C. S., MacIntyre, R. C., Murray, T. A., & Rock, K. Z. (2011). Common themes in clinical education partnerships. *Journal of Nursing Education, 50*(7), 365–372. doi:10.3928/01484834-20110429-01

Trueman, M. S., & Miles, D. G. (2011). Twitter in the classroom: Twenty-first century flash cards. *Nurse Educator, 36*(5), 183–186. Retrieved from http://dx.doi.org/10.1097/NNE.0b013e3182297a07

Tuohy, C. (2011). Collaborative work with industry: Implementation of dedicated education units. *Whitireia Nursing Journal, 18*, 25–38.

U.S. Copyright Office. (2012, June). U.S. fair use guidelines for 17 U.S.C. § 107. Retrieved from http://www.copyright.gov/fls/fl102.html

Upton, D., & Upton, P. (2006). Development of an evidence-based practice questionnaire for nurses. *Journal of Advanced Nursing, 54*, 454–458.

Vitello-Cicciu, J. M. (2002). Exploring emotional intelligence: Implications for nursing leaders. *Journal of Nursing Administration, 32*(4), 203–210.

Vivien, W. X., Tham, L. K., Lau, S., Mei, T. Y., & Kiat, T. K. (2010). An exploration of the critical thinking dispositions of students and their relationship with the preference for simulation as a learning style. *Singapore Nursing Journal, 37*(2), 25–33.

Wagensteen, S., Johansson, I. S., Björkström, M. E., & Nordström, G. (2010). Critical thinking dispositions among newly graduated nurses. *Journal of Advanced Nursing, 66*(10), 2170–2181. Retrieved

from http://dx.doi.org/10.1111/j.1365-2648.2010.05282.x

Wells, M. I., & Dellinger, A. B. (2011). The effect of type of learning environment on perceived learning among graduate nursing students. *Nursing Education Perspectives, 32*(6), 406–410.

Wiggs, C. M. (2010). Collaborative testing: Assessing teamwork and critical thinking behaviors in baccalaureate students. *Nurse Education Today, 31*(3), 279–282. doi:10.1016/j.nedt.2010.10.027

Winters, C. A., & Echeverri, R. (2012). Academic education: Teaching strategies to support evidence-based practice. *Critical Care Nurse, 32*(3), 49–54. Retrieved from http://dx.doi.org/10.4037/ccn2012159

Woith, W., Jenkins, S. D., & Kerber, C. (2012). Perceptions of academic integrity among nursing students. *Nursing Forum, 47*(4), 253–259. Retrieved from http://dx.doi.org/10.1111/j.1744-6198.2012.00274.x

Ziqiong, L., Changrong, C., & Chungping, C. (2012). Study on influence of nurses' emotional intelligence on job burnout [Abstract]. *Chinese Nursing Research, 26*(2A), 310–312.

Zulkowski, A., Ayello, E. A., & Wexler, S. (2007). Certification and education: Do they affect pressure ulcer knowledge in nursing? *Advances in Skin Wound Care, 20*, 34–38.

Zurmehly, J., & Leadingham, C. (2008). Exploring student response systems in nursing education. *CIN: Computers, Informatics, Nursing, 26*(5), 265–270.

Zygmont, D. M., & Schaefer, K. M. (2006). Assessing the critical thinking skills of faculty: What do the findings mean for nursing education? *Nursing Education Perspectives, 27*(5), 260–268.

2

Facilitate Learner Development and Socialization

Susan Luparell, PhD, CNS-BC, CNE

The CNE Test Plan Lists the Following for the Area of Facilitate Learner Development and Socialization:

---

2. Facilitate Learner Development and Socialization

  A. Identify individual learning styles and unique learning needs of learners with these characteristics:

    1. culturally diverse (including international);

    2. English as an additional language

    3. traditional vs. nontraditional (i.e., recent high school graduates vs. those in school later)

    4. at risk (e.g., educationally disadvantaged, learning and/or physically challenged, social, and economic issues)

    5. previous nursing education

  B. Provide resources for diverse learners to meet their individual learning needs

  C. Advise learners in ways that help them meet their professional goals

  D. Create learning environments that facilitate learners' self-reflection, personal goal setting, and socialization to the role of the nurse

  E. Foster the development of learners in these areas:

    1. cognitive domain

    2. psychomotor domain

    3. affective domain

  F. Assist learners to engage in thoughtful and constructive self and peer evaluation

  G. Encourage professional development of learners

The task statements noted in the detailed Certified Nurse Educator test blueprint for Category 2 reflect the nurse educator's role in the important function of facilitating learner development and socialization.

Nurse faculty have many responsibilities related to learner development and socialization. One of the most important functions of the faculty role is to facilitate student transition and socialization into the professional health care environment. Socialization is defined as "a continuing process whereby an individual acquires a personal identity and learns the norms, values, behavior, and social skills appropriate to his or her social position" (Dictionary.com, n.d.); therefore, a new reference to socialization is that of developing a professional identity or formation—transformation of a layperson into a nurse who is able to change "perceptual capacities to act with skilled know-how" (Benner, Sutphen, Leonard, & Day, 2010, p. 166). As part of this transformation, the student must learn not only how to function as a professional nurse on the health care team, but also as a lifelong learner in a rapidly changing health care milieu. Faculty must assist each student to embrace not only nursing but also learning. To best achieve this goal, faculty attend not only to what students learn, but how they learn and how best to meet their unique learning needs. This chapter discusses the role of faculty in facilitating learner development and socialization.

IDENTIFY INDIVIDUAL LEARNING STYLES AND UNIQUE LEARNER NEEDS; PROVIDE RESOURCES FOR DIVERSE LEARNERS TO MEET THEIR INDIVIDUAL LEARNING NEEDS

Learning Styles

Kolb Learning Styles

Kolb (1984; cited in Halstead, 2007) noted that individuals exhibit preferences for how they process information based on two dissecting continuums. A learner tends to process content very concretely, very abstractly, or somewhere in between. Additionally, an individual can take in information in a highly active manner or in a more reflective manner. The combination of these preferences results in four potential learning styles. That is, some students process information with an abstract conceptualization and hands-on active experimentation (convergers). Others process information concretely while reflecting on their observations (divergers). Assimilators have strong inductive reasoning skills and process information using abstract conceptualization and reflective observation. Lastly, some students conceptualize information concretely while employing active experimentation (accommodators). These students are considered hands-on learners. Although students may have patterns and preferences for a particular learning style, learning styles should be considered dynamic, rather than fixed, traits (Kolb & Kolb, 2005).

VARK

Another popular method for categorizing learning styles is by the student's preferred sensory modality with which to take in new information (Wehrwein, Lujan, & DiCarlo, 2007). These sensory preferences rely on different neural systems and include the visual (V), auditory (A), and kinesthetic (K) modes. Fleming (1995) expanded the categories to include a preference for reading or writing (R). Together these four learning preferences are known as VARK.

As the name suggests, visual learners prefer taking in information by sight or observation. Teaching strategies that include demonstrations, diagrams, and pictures often resonate with these learners. Students who are aural learners find live and recorded lectures, as well as discussions, to be useful. R-type learners prefer to interact with words and text in the form of reading and writing. They may take copious notes during class. Finally, kinesthetic learners excel when movement and stimulation of tactile sensation are included in class activities. Hands-on practice and time spent playing with equipment appeal to kinesthetic learners. Although learners use all modalities for inputting information, individuals tend to exhibit unique preferences for one or several modalities. Unimodal learners prefer a single learning style, while multimodal learners prefer using multiple styles (Wehrwein et al., 2007). Dobson (2010) cited several studies suggesting that a majority of physiology students exhibit multimodal preferences; however, it is not clear if this trend holds true for nursing students. Additionally, there are many other factors that can influence learning, including the learning environment, student motivation, and faculty expertise. Nonetheless, the evidence on learning styles and how faculty can best meet the needs of students is emerging, and readers are encouraged to independently review this body of knowledge for a more in-depth understanding.

Identify Needs of a Diverse Student Body

It is becoming clearer that nursing faculty are in many ways fundamentally different from those who make up their classes. In 2009, 93 percent of faculty were over the age of 46, and one in three was over the age of 60 (NLN, 2009). Approximately 86 percent of faculty are white and 95 percent are women (NLN, 2009). Because individuals tend to view the world through their personal framework, these data have important ramifications for how faculty approach learner development. Because student characteristics are often quite different from those of faculty, to best meet the needs of students, faculty must first understand who their students are.

The nursing student body is diverse in many ways. Students in nursing programs represent a wide range of ages with an increasingly greater number of men enrolling. Additionally, the student body is more ethnically and culturally diverse than in previous years. This section examines some key considerations related to the increasingly diverse student body.

Age

The age of students varies across programs, with approximately half of the students enrolled in associate degree in nursing programs under the age of 30 (NLN, 2013), while 74 percent of students in bachelor's degree in nursing programs are under the age of 30.

Traditional students are those who enter college immediately or soon after completing high school. An understanding of what is occurring developmentally with traditional students is helpful for faculty teaching the traditional student. According to Arnett (2004) contemporary young people are in no hurry to reach adulthood. Instead, there is a newly identified life stage between adolescence and adulthood, that of emerging adulthood, which spans the years 18 through 29. A grasp of the primary characteristics of emerging adulthood is useful as faculty assist these young adults to transition into the nursing profession.

There are five key features of emerging adults (Arnett, 2004). Learners in this transitional stage are engaged in *identity exploration*, that is attempting to figure out who they are and what they want out of life. Subsequently, emerging adults may exhibit periods of *instability* marked by frequent changes of jobs, living situations, partners, and so forth. There are periods of *intense self-focus*, sometimes erroneously confused for narcissism, during which the emerging adult is exploring how to qualify for and locate a good job. Students may be reluctant to take on adult responsibilities as they sense a *feeling of being in between*, where they recognize they are no longer adolescents, but do not yet self-identify as fully adult and are, in fact, ambivalent about entering adulthood. Lastly, those transitioning through emerging adulthood tend to have a *sense of possibilities*, recognizing they are on the cusp of a remarkable life and engaging in work they love that hopefully pays well. It is easy to understand that faculty may be befuddled by the behaviors of students transitioning into adulthood. One minute they may espouse wanting to practice as professional nurses, while the next minute they may appear unable to take responsibility for their learning.

Not all students are traditional. Students and faculty in nursing classrooms may represent multiple generations with a number of cohorts of individuals born in roughly the same timeframe who have similar experiences and frames of reference. Thus, they tend to share values, attitudes, expectations, and motivational stimuli (Hammill, 2005), which is effective as educators plan educational activities to meet the needs of generationally diverse students.

Most faculty fall into the baby boomer generation (NLN, 2013), identified as those born between 1946 and 1964 (Hammill, 2005). Baby boomers tend to have a strong work ethic and value the quality of their work. They value personal communication (Gibson, 2009). Conversely, most students are classified as members of Generation X or Generation Y. Generation Xers, born between 1965 and 1980, tend to see all people as part of the same peer group, feel free to challenge authority, are task-oriented, feel constrained by rules (Gibson, 2009), and seek immediate gratification (Hammill, 2005). Generation Y includes those born between 1981 and 2000. Traditional college students belong to Generation Y and are sometimes referred to as millennials (Hammill, 2005). Millennials view education as a means to an end, are team- and goal-oriented, perceive themselves as multitaskers, and prefer to communicate via email or text (Hammill, 2005).

To decrease conflict in the classroom and meet the needs of various age groups, faculty understand the attitudes and values associated with the various generations but avoid broad sweeping generalizations. Teaching strategies and communication are geared toward the generational preferences of the students. For example, Generation Xers prefer directions that are concise and to the point and want immediate feedback on their work (Gibson, 2009). Millennials may learn best in group activities and appreciate the use of text message blasts to communicate important changes in schedules.

Ethnic, Cultural, and Social Diversity

Although the percentage of minority students has risen from the early 1990s, it has remained fairly stable over the past several years (NLN, 2013). As of fall 2012, approximately one in four nursing students identified themselves as a minority. African Americans represent the highest percentage of minority students (12.9 percent), followed by Hispanic students (6.8 percent), and Asian or Pacific Island students (5.6 percent). Still, the makeup of minorities in nursing programs is not equivalent to the minority representation among all U.S. college students.

Culture is a representation of values, habits, and beliefs acquired over time as a member of a group. It is important to remember that culture is not solely tied to ethnicity, and all individuals belong to multiple groups. Increasingly nurse educators identify students who are first-generation college students or represent various socioeconomic backgrounds, family structures, or regions of the country. Even being from a rural versus an urban area influences a student's particular approach to learning. Faculty assess the unique influences of culture on student learning needs and plan their teaching accordingly.

English as an Additional Language

Students who know English not as their primary but as an additional language represent a further subset of the minority student population. The terms English language learners (ELL) and English as a second language (ESL) are also used when referring to this group of students. These students speak two or more languages and may be international or immigrant learners (Olson, 2012). Faculty should also bear in mind that a student may appear to be an English speaker and perhaps was even born in the United States but may have been raised in a home where the primary language was not English. These students may ostensibly speak English quite well, but may actually think and process ideas in an alternative language, which may manifest itself in the form of subtle communication challenges or test-taking difficulties.

Historically, ESL students experience unique challenges during their nursing education, most of which stem from language difficulties. For instance, these students may have a difficult time understanding medical terminology or communicating with patients and staff. Subsequently, there is a higher rate of attrition among ELS students with a collectively lower National Council Licensure Examination pass rate than that of native speakers (Olson, 2012). Following a comprehensive literature review, Olson (2012) discovered that mixing study groups with both ESL and native speakers consistently appeared to facilitate language skills. Additionally, audio recording class sessions and providing copies of class materials may prove helpful for ESL students. Engaging ESL students in role-playing activities in which they practice interacting with patients and staff may further facilitate communication skills and relieve anxiety.

Not all challenges faced by ESL students are related to language. International or immigrant students may experience significant conflicts between their own cultural background and the American educational and health care systems (Olson, 2012). Additionally, ESL students may find themselves to be victims of racism and other stereotyping by fellow students, faculty, agency staff, and patients. To minimize barriers based on culture, faculty work to create a climate of openness, value, and respect.

Gender Diversity

Although the number of men in nursing school outpaces the working nurse population (9.6 percent) (U.S. Department of Health and Human Services, 2010), nursing students are overwhelmingly women (85 percent) across all program types (NLN, 2013). The evidence is equivocal on whether there are learning style differences based on gender. For example, when comparing VARK learning styles among male and female medical students in India, no differences were found between the genders, and both genders overwhelmingly preferred multimodal learning engaging all the senses (Kumar, Smriti, Pratap, & Krishnee, 2012). However, researchers found significant differences in learning styles among American men and women physiology students (Wehrwein et al., 2007), with 87.5 percent of the men but only 45.8 percent of the women preferring to take in information by multiple modes. ? Why?

Students with Previous Education

There has been a burgeoning of accelerated nursing programs in recent years, into which are enrolled adult students who have already obtained a college degree in another field. These students choose to enter nursing for a variety of reasons, including a desire to follow through on a previous interest or acquire stable employment. They tend to have diverse characteristics, most notably in terms of background and experience, and many have multiple responsibilities outside of school (Siler, DeBasio, & Roberts, 2008). Additionally, accelerated students may experience unique financial issues. Because accelerated programs are more time intensive than traditional programs, students often hold part-time jobs or may have no employment and may not be eligible for grant and scholarship opportunities afforded first-time students (Siler et al., 2008).

Evidence suggests that accelerated students desire different teaching approaches for success. Based on the characteristics of this group of learners, strategies that

But the Indian education system is one-size-fits-all!

can facilitate student success include experiential learning, self-directed learning, and those based on the social-cognitive theory of learning (Johnson, 2010). In particular, faculty should consider employing teaching strategies that provide students the opportunity to assimilate their new nursing knowledge with previous experiences.

At-Risk Students

Many factors can deem a student to be at risk for failing a nursing program. Students who are economically or academically disadvantaged may be at risk. Factors that can predispose a student to being at risk are many and varied, but they can be grouped according to academic factors, personal factors, and environmental factors. Box 2.1 presents a listing of these factors. Positive factors affecting retention have also been identified (see Box 2.2).

Faculty must identify the at-risk characteristics within their student body. A yearly analysis is helpful because characteristics of students can change over the years. Once identified, faculty can plan interventions to assist students with the various factors impacting their ability to complete the nursing program. Completion

---

BOX 2.1 At-Risk Factors

Academic Factors
Test anxiety and test taking
Difficulty with critical thinking
Low level of reading comprehension
Poor note-taking ability
Personal feelings about studying and school
Feelings of loneliness; isolation in the school setting
Difficulty coping with amount of coursework
Dissatisfaction with program requirements
Inadequate preparation for coursework
Transportation; traveling distance

Personal Factors
Personal feelings about college
Attitude toward attendance
Attitude toward study skills
Lack of preentrance counseling
Non-English language background
Poor time management
Poor stress management
Low level of motivation
Lack of perseverance
Lack of self-confidence; low self-esteem
Health problems

Environmental Factors
Too many hours of employment
Financial difficulties
Heavy job obligations
Family, too many home responsibilities
Family problems
Overly committed to church, community activities

Adapted with permission from Caputi and Engelmann (2008).

BOX 2.2 Positive Factors Impacting Retention of Nursing Students

Academic Factors
Collaborative learning environment
Good student-to-faculty rapport
Faculty guidance and support
Frequent student-faculty interaction

Personal Factors
Recognition of personal worth
Motivation

Environmental Factors
Formal campus learning activities
Social support system
Study groups
Good student-to-student rapport
Involvement with campus activities *But not too much*

Adapted with permission from Caputi and Engelmann (2008).

---

rates are critical for the students but also for the program. Many accreditation agencies to whom the nursing programs are accountable use retention rate as a measure of a quality program.

Students with a Disability

The Americans with Disabilities Act (ADA) of 1990 requires that students with certain types of physical or mental illnesses or other disabilities be afforded reasonable accommodations to meet course and program requirements (U.S. Equal Employment Opportunity Commission, 2008). For example, a student with a hearing impairment may require an audio-enhanced stethoscope or a student with a learning disability may require additional time to complete exams. Once the system is accessed, specialized personnel assist the faculty to identify appropriate student accommodations and discuss individualized learning strategies. Students who receive accommodations must ultimately meet individual course requirements in order to successfully move forward. Faculty are encouraged to speak with the ADA officers at their own institutions to become more familiar with this important legislation and specific implications for nursing education.

The ADA mandates that no qualified individual with a disability can, because of the disability, be denied participation in or the benefit of services, programs, or activities of a public entity, place of public accommodation, or other covered entity. In this way the ADA protects the rights of individuals with disabilities enrolled in an educational program. Students with disabilities are guaranteed equal access to a nursing education if they are otherwise qualified (Christensen, 2010).

Not all disabilities covered by the ADA are specifically named. General physical disabilities covered include both physical disabilities such as those who are hearing impaired or visually impaired or diagnosed with a chronic illness. Mental disabilities are also covered, such as attention deficit disorder, learning disability, or a mood disorder (Christensen, 2010).

The law states that otherwise qualified individuals may not be denied admission solely on the basis of a disability. Additionally, admission criteria cannot be used that has the effect of discriminating against handicapped individuals. The phrase "otherwise qualified" is key. Generally, otherwise qualified means the individual can, with adaptations or accommodations, perform the duties or requirements as required for that educational program. Because of this, higher education institutions must make reasonable accommodations for students with disabilities. While providing reasonable accommodations, the nursing program is not required to substantially change the course of study or lower academic standards. The educational institution is not required to make accommodations that result in undue hardship for the school. The cost of the accommodations is placed on the educational institution (when receiving federal financial assistance). If providing the needed assistance causes an undue burden, then the school is not required to provide the accommodation (Christensen, 2010).

Additionally, the student must ask for the accommodation. This means the student must disclose the disability and ask for the accommodations. The school then can require documentation or evaluation of the student to verify the exact type of disability and the most reasonable accommodation for the situation. Therefore, the student cannot ask for accommodations without the requested accommodation recommended by a professional who has evaluated the student (Christensen, 2010).

ADVISE LEARNERS TO ASSIST IN MEETING PROFESSIONAL GOALS

Advising is another important aspect of the faculty role and has been shown to have a positive influence on retention and other measures of student success (Trent, 1997). Conceptually, the advising role can be approached from a prescriptive or developmental point of view. Gasper (2009) noted that prescriptive advising generally involves simple answering of concrete student questions, while developmental advising incorporates personalized guidance designed to assist the student in managing both academic and general life concerns. Prescriptive advising requires a thorough understanding of the program curriculum as well as institutional policies. Developmental advising focuses on fostering a student's decision-making skills while helping the student assume responsibility for those decisions. For example, an adviser could assist a student to consider the pros and cons of taking an additional elective. Additionally, faculty are often in a position to help students assess unique strengths and help identify what nursing role will best match the identified skill set. Alternatively, if a student feels strongly about a professional goal, faculty can help the student focus on specific needs or improvements that will assist in achieving the goal.

Gasper (2009, p. 90) describes the role of adviser as that of "supportive critic." To foster student development and decision-making, the adviser must be skilled at building rapport, listening, problem solving, and interviewing. Additionally, the adviser must respect and value students as individuals, be open to their opinions, and have genuine concern for their growth and well-being. Lastly, the adviser must treat nondirectory student information with confidentiality as mandated by the Family Education Rights and Privacy Act (U.S. Department of Education, 2011).

CREATE LEARNING ENVIRONMENTS TO FOSTER LEARNER DEVELOPMENT

In terms of general approaches to teaching and learning, many nurse educators draw on Kolb's Experiential Learning Theory (ELT) to guide their work. Consistent

Like Mezirow!

with his belief that "learning is the major process of human adaptation" (Kolb, 1984, p. 32), there are six propositions to ELT (Kolb, 1984; Kolb & Kolb, 2005):

Kolb's experiential learning theory

1. Learning is more of a process than a set of outcomes.
2. Learning occurs as students examine and redefine their values and beliefs in light of new ideas.
3. Disagreement among ideas drives the learning process.
4. Learning is a process of adaptation to the world involving changes in one's thinking, perceiving, and behaving.
5. Learning involves transactions during which new experiences are assimilated into existing concepts or existing concepts are understood in the context of new experiences.
6. Learning is a process whereby knowledge is actually constructed by the student as opposed to merely transmitting fixed ideas from teacher to student.

According to ELT, educators focus not only on the content of the learning, but also on the processes of learning, including how students engage in learning. Additionally, faculty who apply experiential learning theory as they develop teaching strategies encourage students to consider how new content fits contextually with their past experiences as well as how their past experiences influence the new learning.

FOSTER LEARNER DEVELOPMENT IN THREE DOMAINS OF LEARNING

Bloom's Taxonomy identified three domains toward which learning activities are directed. The original taxonomy has been subsequently revised and enhanced (Anderson & Krathwohl, 2001), although the original version is often cited. Each domain includes a series of developmental levels, or hierarchies, to be achieved, starting with the most basic functions of the domain and moving toward the more complex. For example, in the cognitive domain, remembering is the most basic function and requires the learner to recall knowledge of facts, not necessarily related to any specific context. Student learning outcomes are written at higher cognitive levels as the courses build throughout the program. Therefore, the level of students' thinking progresses as they achieve the higher-level course student learning outcomes. The nurse educator plans teaching and learning activities that challenge students to attain the higher levels of functioning in each of these domains as they progress throughout the program.

Cognitive Domain

The cognitive domain addresses thinking at six progressively more complex levels of sophistication. At the most basic level, students *remember* factual information. As students develop in the cognitive domain, activities challenge students to think at higher cognitive levels. Thinking progresses to the ability to *understand* the meaning of information and *apply* it to relevant scenarios. Teachers then guide students as they *analyze* and *evaluate* information. At the highest level of cognitive function, students *create* new meanings and experiences. It is generally presumed that students move up the hierarchy in a somewhat linear fashion. That is, students cannot *apply* information on potassium levels if they do not first *understand* factual information such as the normal levels of potassium and what potassium regulates.

To best foster student development, the faculty are cognizant of the ultimate goal and create activities that promote advancement through the hierarchy of cognitive learning. For example, flash cards may help students learn important medical terms at the remember level of proficiency. Well-developed case studies require the student to analyze information in the context of the study. Alternatively, development of a concept map linking the relationship between immune function, sleep, and nutrition requires the student to understand the most important concepts of each and create a product that visually portrays the linkages.

Psychomotor Domain

When providing nursing care it is important for the nurse to safely and competently perform a nursing skill. The psychomotor domain addresses the development of motor skills. Levels of complexity range from observing and imitating to fine tuning and adapting to unique situations (Bixler, n.d.). For example, at higher levels of functioning in the psychomotor domain, a student is able to adapt a skill based on the specific type of equipment available or based on a patient's unique needs. As a general rule, frequent repetition is a prerequisite of skills proficiency, and faculty should consider factoring in opportunities for ongoing practice during course and curriculum planning.

Affective Domain = beliefs values emotional

The affective domain is associated with attitudes, beliefs, values, and emotions and is especially important for the development of ethical comportment and professional formation espoused by Benner and colleagues (2010). As with the other domains, the affective domain is also associated with an increasing level of achievement, ranging from simple acknowledgment of a belief or value to its full embodiment demonstrated by how one lives and carries on (Bixler, n.d.). To effectively address the affective domain, the nurse educator develops teaching strategies and learning activities that stimulate an emotional response or cause a student to reconsider values and beliefs. For example, a class debate exposing two sides of an ethical issue may cause intrapersonal conflict resulting in critical introspection about what one believes and why.

ASSIST LEARNERS TO ENGAGE IN CONSTRUCTIVE EVALUATION OF SELF AND OTHERS

An important component of professional maturity is the ability to thoughtfully and constructively analyze performance and provide feedback to facilitate improvement. This process must occur at both the individual and team levels. To enhance the learner's ability to engage in self-evaluation, faculty include opportunities for students to do so.

Providing realistic and honest feedback, while not being intentionally hurtful, is a skill that will be useful to students in the workplace. Faculty should incorporate opportunities for students to learn this skill and frequently remind students of the beneficial influence that honest self-appraisal plays in role development. Examples include self-reflection journals and guided introspection. Additionally, faculty can role model providing constructive feedback in their dealings with students. A trusting relationship is essential when providing feedback (Luparell, 2007). Students are reminded that the motive for sharing constructive feedback is to help the student succeed and flourish in the nursing role. Activities in which students must provide feedback to their peers may also be useful to enhance interpersonal skills.

ENCOURAGE PROFESSIONAL DEVELOPMENT

In addition to helping students acquire the requisite knowledge and skills for safe and effective nursing practice, faculty are called upon to help develop ethical comportment and formation (Benner et al., 2010). Adequate socialization involves helping students realize and accept the full breadth of what is expected of nurses, including the values, morals, and attitudes espoused by the profession.

An important topic in today's educational environment is that of incivility in nursing and nursing education. Initial interest in incivility in nursing education came from the perspective of faculty frustration with misbehaving students (Clark & Springer, 2007; Luparell, 2004). More recently, however, concern has been expressed that students are negatively socialized to proper interpersonal communication during their formative years (Luparell, 2011), and there are numerous reports of students' experiences with incivility from both faculty and agency staff (Clark, 2008; Lasiter, Marchiondo, & Marchiondo, 2012; Thomas & Burk, 2009).

The prevalence of horizontal violence, in which practicing nurses treat one another with a fundamental lack of respect, has been well documented. Only recently, however, are the true ramifications of incivility and disruptive behavior in the health care environment being realized. For example, the psychological and physical impact on nurses' health has been reported in response to disruptive behavior (Dumont, Meisinger, Whitacre, & Corbin, 2012; Rosenstein & O'Daniel, 2005; Vessey, Demarco, & DiFazio, 2010). Furthermore, workplace incivility has been linked to decreased nurse productivity (Hutton & Gates, 2008) and decreased job satisfaction (Vessey et al., 2010). Most importantly, injury, death, and other negative patient outcomes have been linked to incivility and disruptive behavior among the health care team (Rosenstein & O'Daniel, 2005). Therefore, in terms of socialization, the ethical imperatives to graduate nurses who improve the work environment rather than detract from it are significant.

To best facilitate development of ethical comportment, especially as it relates to interpersonal interactions within the profession, faculty should make civility in their classrooms a priority. Students need to clearly understand the behavioral expectations and why these expectations are important to patient safety. Additionally, faculty themselves, as role models of the profession, must embrace civility in their interactions with students and with one another.

SUMMARY

This chapter has covered many areas related to facilitating learner development and socialization. Additional topics you may want to review include the following:

- Novice to expert theory: novice, advanced beginner, competency, proficient, expert
- Specific strategies to foster the cognitive domain including:
  - Debates
  - Cooperative or collaborative learning

- Unfolding case studies
- Problem-based learning
- Formal written assignments such as research critiques and focused writings
- Portfolios
- Levels of development of the affective domain: receiving, responding, valuing, organizing, internalizing
- Student cheating
- Phases of Kramer's Reality Shock: honeymoon, shock/rejection, recovery, resolution

Although the most visible aspect of teaching is to share knowledge and expertise with students, the role is both much more complex and much more subtle. Faculty have profound influence over student development on many levels. For students to maximize their potential, the learning environment must be one in which students perceive they are free to explore ideas and try new approaches without undue criticism. To best facilitate learning, faculty are charged with understanding their students both collectively and as individuals. Only after gaining such insight can faculty fully address student learning needs.

Practice Test Questions

1. Which strategy will the nurse educator use to teach a group of adult learners?
   A. Develop learning experiences that build on previous experiences and learning
   B. Provide highly structured learning activities that limit individualization of learning
   C. Avoid the use of teaching strategies that foster reflective practice
   D. Minimize learner participation when identifying individual learning needs

2. The nursing faculty expects students in a pathophysiology course to correlate physiological changes experienced by patients with complex medical problems to their clinical status. Which strategy will the instructor choose to best facilitate this analysis?
   A. Algorithms
   B. Clinical simulation
   C. Concept mapping
   D. One-minute paper

3. A fourth-year baccalaureate nursing student is having difficulty inserting intravenous catheters and is not demonstrating aseptic technique. This skill was taught in a previous course. What action will the instructor initiate to best rectify this situation?
   A. Fail the student in the course for not mastering this skill
   B. Assign a short paper on how to maintain aseptic technique during catheterization
   C. Refer the student to the nursing lab instructor for coaching and practice
   D. Have the student reflect on strengths and weaknesses in the clinical area in the weekly journal

4. A nurse educator is attempting to address various learning styles when delivering didactic contact. Which approach will best facilitate this endeavor?
   A. Develop at least one classroom activity that meets the needs of each representative learning style
   B. Assign group classroom activities for which each group is composed of students with different learning styles
   C. Communicate to students that completion of classroom activities will provide the necessary tools for success
   D. Provide classroom activities that encourage faculty-student interaction

5. Which student learning outcome best represents the affective domain of learning? The student will:
   A. Develop basic plans of care utilizing the nursing process for patients with common alterations in health status
   B. Conduct an initial physical assessment of a patient with common health-related interference in functional health patterns
   C. Respond to aspects of sociocultural influences that impact the health of families
   D. Identify and apply relevant principles of pathophysiology related to alterations in metabolism

(continued on page 46)

6. Which strategy would be most beneficial to facilitate learning for ESL students?
   A. Provide individual tutoring sessions especially for the ESL students
   B. Require ESL students to take additional English language classes
   C. Require ESL students to complete assignments both in writing and orally
   D. Organize team-based learning strategies that partner ESL and native English speakers

7. To meet the needs of students who have a preference for kinesthetic learning, an instructor should employ which strategy?
   A. Allow taping of lectures
   B. Provide hands-on activities during class
   C. Provide handouts that require students to fill in and take notes
   D. Incorporate short periods of quiet time for reading during class

8. The instructor who draws on experiential learning theory would use which principle in course planning?
   A. How students go about learning requires as much attention as what they are learning.
   B. Students need to share common experiences to form a sense of community.
   C. Students will need to shed their understanding of previous life experiences.
   D. New modes of learning will be required to teach students with diverse backgrounds.

9. Which is the primary reason for ensuring appropriate student behavior and ethical comportment is addressed in the nursing program of study?
   A. Maintain control of the classroom
   B. Preserve the image of the profession
   C. Facilitate learning
   D. Ensure patient safety

10. Which implication is true regarding the American with Disabilities Act?
    A. The faculty member is responsible for identifying a student's disability and providing accommodations.
    B. Students with disabilities must be able to perform the essential functions of the nursing student role.
    C. A school must expend all efforts to ensure accommodations are provided.
    D. Evaluation of students with disabilities is performed using a different set of criteria from other students.

References

Anderson, L. W., & Krathwohl, D. R. (Eds.). (2001). *A taxonomy for learning, teaching and assessing: A revision of Bloom's Taxonomy of educational objectives: Complete edition.* New York: Longman.

Arnett, J. J. (2004). *Emerging adulthood: The winding road from the late teens through the twenties.* New York: Oxford University Press.

Benner, P., Sutphen, M., Leonard, V., & Day, L. (2010). *Educating nurses: A call for radical transformation.* San Francisco: Jossey-Bass.

Bixler, B. (n.d.). The ABCDs of writing instructional objectives. Retrieved from http://www.personal. psu.edu/bxb11/Objectives/ActionVerbsfor Objectives.pdf

Caputi, L., & Engelmann, L. (2008). *Teaching nursing: The art and science, volume 4, it's all about student success.* Glen Ellyn, IL: College of DuPage Press.

Christensen, L. (2010). The law and disabilities: How the ADA affects nursing education. In L. Caputi (Ed.), *Teaching nursing: The art and science, volume 3.* Glen Ellyn, IL: College of DuPage Press.

Clark, C. (2008). Student perspectives on faculty incivility in nursing education: An application of the concept of rankism. *Nursing Outlook, 56*(1), 4.

Clark, C., & Springer, P. (2007). Thoughts on incivility: Student and faculty perceptions of uncivil behavior in nursing education. *Nursing Education Perspectives, 28*(2), 93–97.

Dobson, J. A. (2010). A comparison between learning style preferences and sex, status, and course performance. *Advances in Physiology Education, 34*(4), 197–204.

Dumont, C., Meisinger, S., Whitacre, M. J., & Corbin, G. (2012). Horizontal violence survey report. *Nursing, 42*(1), 44–49.

Fleming, N. D. (1995). *I'm different; not dumb.* Modes of presentation (VARK) in the tertiary classroom. In A. Zelmer (Ed.), *Research and development in higher education. Proceedings of the 1995 Annual Conference of the Higher Education and Research Development Society of Australasia, 18*, 308–313.

Gasper, M. (2009). Building a community with your advisees. *Nurse Educator, 34*(2), 88–94.

Gibson, S. E. (2009). Intergenerational communication in the classroom: Recommendations for successful teacher-student relationships. *Nursing Education Perspectives, 30*(1), 37–39.

Halstead, J. A. (Ed.). (2007). *Nurse educator competencies: Creating an evidence-based practice for nurse educators.* New York: National League for Nursing.

Hammill, G. (2005, Winter/Spring). Mixing and managing four generations of employees. Retrieved from http://www.fdu.edu/newspubs/magazine/05ws/generations.htm

Hutton, S., & Gates, D. (2008). Workplace incivility and productivity losses among direct care staff. *AAOHN Journal, 56*(4), 168.

Johnson, L. (2010). *How accelerated nursing students learn: A comparative case study of the facilitators, barriers, learning strategies, challenges, and obstacles of students in an accelerated nursing program.* Unpublished doctoral dissertation. Teachers College, Columbia University.

Kolb, D. A. (1984). *Experiential learning: Experiences as the source of learning and development.* Englewood Cliffs, NJ: Prentice-Hall.

Kolb, A. Y., & Kolb, D. A. (2005). Learning styles and learning spaces: Enhancing experiential learning in higher education. *Academy of Management Learning & Education, 4*(2), 193–212.

Kumar, A., Smriti, A., Pratap, S., & Krishnee, G. (2012). An analysis of gender differences in learning style preferences among medical students. *Indian Journal of Forensic Medicine & Pathology, 5*(1), 9–16.

Lasiter, S., Marchiondo, L., & Marchiondo, K. (2012). Student narratives of faculty incivility. *Nursing Outlook, 60*(3), 121.

Luparell, S. (2004). Faculty encounters with uncivil nursing students: An overview. *Journal of Professional Nursing, 20*(1), 59–67.

Luparell, S. (2007). Dealing with challenging student situations: Lessons learned. In M. H. Oermann & K. T. Heinrich (Eds.), *Annual review of nursing education: Vol. 5. Challenges and new directions in nursing education* (pp. 101-110). New York: Springer.

Luparell, S. (2011). Incivility in nursing: The connection between academia and the workplace. *Critical Care Nurse, 31*(2), 92–95.

National League for Nursing (NLN). (2009). Faculty census. NLN DataView™. Retrieved from http://www.nln.org/research/slides/index.htm

National League for Nursing (NLN). (2013). Annual review of nursing schools. NLN DataView™. Retrieved from http://www.nln.org/research/slides/index.htm

Olson, M. (2012). English-as-a-second language (ESL) nursing student success: A critical review of the literature. *Journal of Cultural Diversity, 19*(1), 26–32.

Rosenstein, A. H., & O'Daniel, M. (2005). Disruptive behavior & clinical outcomes: Perceptions of nurses & physicians. *American Journal of Nursing, 105*(1), 54–64.

Siler, B., DeBasio, N., & Roberts, K. (2008). Profile of non-nurse college graduates enrolled in accelerated baccalaureate curricula: Results of a national study. *Nursing Education Perspectives, 29*(6), 336–341.

Thomas, S. P., & Burk, R. (2009). Junior nursing students' experiences of vertical violence during clinical rotations. *Nursing Outlook, 57*(4), 226.

Trent, B. (1997). Student perceptions of academic advising in an RN-to-BSN program. *Journal of Continuing Education In Nursing, 28*(6), 276–283.

U.S. Department of Education. (2011). Family Educational Rights and Privacy Act (FERPA). Retrieved from http://www2.ed.gov/policy/gen/guid/fpco/ferpa/students.html

U.S. Department of Health and Human Services. (2010, Winter). The registered nurse population: Findings from the 2008 National Sample Survey of Registered Nurses. Retrieved from http://bhpr.hrsa.gov/healthworkforce/rnsurveys/rnsurveyfinal.pdf

U.S. Equal Employment Opportunity Commission. (2008). Facts about the Americans with Disabilities Act. Retrieved from http://www.eeoc.gov/facts/fs-ada.html

Vessey, J. A., Demarco, R., & DiFazio, R. (2010). Bullying, harassment, and horizontal violence in the nursing workforce: The state of the science. *Annual Review of Nursing Research, 28*, 133–157. doi:10.1891/0739-6686.28.133

Wehrwein, E. A., Lujan, H. L., & DiCarlo, S. E. (2007). Gender differences in learning style preferences among undergraduate physiology students. *Advances in Physiology Education, 31*, 153–157. doi:10.1152/advan.00060.2006

3

Use Assessment and Evaluation Strategies

Gail Baumlein, PhD, RN, CNS, CNE, ANEF

The CNE Test Plan Lists the Following for the Area of Use Assessment and Evaluation Strategies:

3. Use Assessment and Evaluation Strategies

A. Provide input for the development of nursing program standards and policies regarding:
  1. admission
  2. progression
  3. graduation
B. Enforce nursing program standards related to:
  1. admission
  2. progression
  3. graduation
C. Use a variety of strategies to assess and evaluate learning in these domains:
  1. cognitive
  2. psychomotor
  3. affective
D. Incorporate current research in assessment and evaluation practices
E. Analyze available resources for learner assessment and evaluation
F. Create assessment instruments to evaluate outcomes
G. Use assessment instruments to evaluate outcomes
H. Implement evaluation strategies that are appropriate to the learner and learning outcomes
I. Analyze assessment and evaluation data
J. Use assessment and evaluation data to enhance the teaching-learning process
K. Advise learners regarding assessment and evaluation criteria
L. Provide timely, constructive, and thoughtful feedback to learners

The National League for Nursing (NLN) Certified Nurse Educator test plan Category 3 focuses on assessment and evaluation. Nurse educators use a multitude of strategies to assess and evaluate student learning. To maximize the effectiveness of these strategies, nurse educators:

- Use extant literature to develop evidence-based assessment and evaluation practices
- Use a variety of strategies to assess and evaluate learning in the cognitive, psychomotor, and affective domains
- Implement evidence-based assessment and evaluation strategies that are appropriate to the learner and to learning goals
- Use assessment and evaluation data to enhance the teaching-learning process
- Provide timely, constructive, and thoughtful feedback to learners
- Demonstrate skill in the design and use of tools for assessing clinical practice (NLN, 2012b, p. 17).

USE ASSESSMENT AND EVALUATION DATA TO ENHANCE THE TEACHING-LEARNING PROCESS; INCORPORATE CURRENT RESEARCH IN ASSESSMENT AND EVALUATION PRACTICES

Nurse educators are accountable for using evidence-based assessment and evaluation methods in classroom and clinical settings to maintain the quality of educational programs. Incorporating current research in assessment and evaluation practices provides a strong foundation for enhancing the teaching-learning process. Research evidence in empirical literature, white papers, position statements, and education-related references can help faculty develop relevant assessment and evaluation strategies. For example, the *NLN Fair Testing Imperative in Nursing Education* provides guidelines for use of standardized testing in assessment (NLN, 2012a). Reading current publications on developing assessment methods is essential for developing valid and reliable examinations and other assessment methods.

Teachers select appropriate strategies to assess achievement of learning in the cognitive, psychomotor, and affective domains, while also using assessment and evaluation data to inform decisions about courses, programs, and curricula. These data are also used in determining educational standards such as admission, progression, and graduation policies (Oermann & Gaberson, 2009).

Given the central nature of assessment and evaluation to nursing education, this chapter begins with a clarification of the definitions of these two terms. *Assessment* refers to measures that provide information about students' abilities before, during, and after participation in programs (Billings & Halstead, 2012). Assessment includes both qualitative and quantitative data, which are used to provide feedback for students about their performance, as well as information and data for the educator to use in determining whether students have met the student learning outcomes and competencies. Educators rely on assessment data to improve educational practices, strengthen programs, and develop educational policies.

The process of assessment is ongoing throughout the teaching-learning cycle. Assessment is used prior to developing programs, outcomes, and instructional methods. Preadmission testing is one means of assessment used to determine levels of students' needs and helps inform the development of the program and the courses. Teachers modify instruction based on feedback attained through assessment of student learning. Figure 3.1 depicts this continuous and circular process.

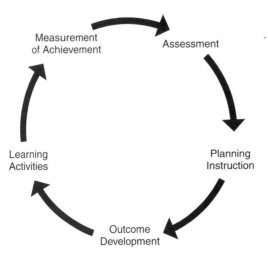

FIGURE 3.1 Interaction of Assessment in Planning, Outcome Development, Learning Strategies, Measuring Achievement.

Sometimes the word *measurement* is used interchangeably with the word *assessment*; it is not, however, synonymous. *Measurement* is a process of assigning numbers to represent student performance or achievement (Oermann & Gaberson, 2009). For example, a test score is a means for measuring the degree of student learning. Key to understanding this concept is recognizing that the ability to interpret measurement scores requires a frame of reference. Comparing one student's score or performance with others in a group, or *norm referencing*, answers the question, How well do they compare with others? Although grading on a curve is a much-used form of norm referencing and can provide worthwhile assessment data, a disadvantage of this method is that it does not provide a means to judge student achievement in relationship to outcomes.

In contrast, *criterion referencing* interprets scores based on preset criteria, rather than on comparison with other students. This is sometimes referred to as *competency-based measurement,* where achievement of a defined set of competencies measures student learning. For example, exam scores represent a criterion-referenced interpretation of student performance. Evaluation of performance of psychomotor skills often uses a criterion-referenced tool, such as a checklist or rubric, to grade specific behaviors associated with the skill.

The second concept central to this discussion is *evaluation.* Although myriad definitions address *evaluation,* in a basic sense, evaluating something means appraising its quality. Educational evaluation usually refers to a systematic appraisal of the quality of education. Because educators are accountable for evaluating the quality of the education they deliver, they are expected to use formal processes to perform a systematic evaluation of numerous areas, including student achievement of outcomes. To do so, educators use two major types of evaluation—*formative* and *summative*—and both are used in nursing programs. *Formative evaluation* occurs throughout the process of instruction and provides feedback about students' progress, with a goal of improving learning and improving clinical competency (Oermann & Gaberson, 2009). Formative evaluation allows teachers to continually assess student learning and enables them to provide specific feedback about student performance, as well as improve teaching strategies, the course, or the curriculum. During clinical instruction, teachers engage in ongoing observations used to guide the students' performance. Teachers can make immediate changes in instruction based on formative evaluation feedback, thus allowing students to modify their performance to achieve student learning outcomes.

Summative evaluation occurs at the end of instruction and determines the overall achievement of the student in the course or at the end of the program. In essence, summative evaluation *sums up* or *summarizes* the outcome of the education. The final grade in a course is an example of summative evaluation, but other examples of methods used for summative evaluation include exams, capstone projects and written assignments, portfolios, and practicum exams.

Program evaluation is an absolutely essential component of ensuring quality in education. Teachers conduct assessment and evaluation activities continuously to improve learning, student outcomes, and program quality. Schools generally develop a lengthy systematic plan for evaluation that designates what will be evaluated, what assessments measures are used, who is responsible for completing the evaluation or gathering the data, when components are evaluated, and how results are reported. Regulatory agencies such as the state board of nursing or state higher education boards, as well as nursing discipline accrediting bodies, examine a school's evaluation plan to determine if all aspects of the educational experience are evaluated and whether the results are being used for ongoing curricula and program improvement. The nurse educator is integral in the evaluation process and should be knowledgeable of the many elements of the school's evaluation plan.

PROVIDE INPUT FOR THE DEVELOPMENT OF NURSING PROGRAM STANDARDS AND POLICIES; ENFORCE NURSING PROGRAM STANDARDS

Educators are often called upon by their school's administration to provide input into student policies for admission, progression, and graduation. Basing these policies and decisions on relevant evidence supports high-quality education and student outcomes.

Admission Policies

Admission policies typically include a series of basic requirements, such as:

1. Graduation from an approved or accredited program that provides the basic foundation for the program (i.e., graduation from high school for a student seeking admission to a prelicensure nursing program)
2. A minimum required GPA in previous education
3. A minimum score on a standardized entry examination
4. Ability to read and write English if it is not the native language of the applicant
5. Submission of official transcripts
6. Relevant prerequisites such as an RN license for registered nurse applicants seeking admission to a registered nursing bachelor's or graduate nursing program.

Some requirements, such as verification of completion of programs by providing official transcripts and proof of RN licensure, may be mandated by regulatory agencies such as boards of nursing, accrediting bodies, and higher education boards.

The nurse educator may be part of a committee that determines admission policies or approves applicants for admission. The purpose of these policies is to create meaningful criteria that facilitate the selection and approval processes, ultimately enabling admissions officials to determine which applicants are the most qualified and most likely to graduate. Standardized tests can play a role in determining an applicant's eligibility for admission, as schools attempt to predict ultimate success, especially on the National Council Licensure Examination for Registered Nurses (NCLEX-RN®). Standardized tests, such as the ACT, SAT, or GRE, or nursing-specific entrance exams, such as the Test of Essential Academic Skills (TEAS) and the Nurse Entrance Test (NET), are often used to establish a baseline for admission. It is important, however, to consider empirical evidence when considering a preadmission testing policy, as limited data are available to support these exams as predictors of success in coursework or on the NCLEX-RN (Frank, 2010).

Progression Policies

Schools have policies that regulate progression within a program. For example, a policy may state a student must achieve a minimum grade of C in a nursing course to progress to the next nursing course or to graduation. The minimum grade earned in nursing courses required for progression is often higher than for nonnursing courses. Most nursing programs require a grade of C while other non-nursing courses allow progression with a D grade. Additionally, the grading scale for nursing—that is the percentages earned for an A, B, or C—is typically higher than for nonnursing courses. Additional data for prelicensure nursing programs used to determine progression include satisfactory performance in clinical, grades on a dosage calculation examination, and successful performance of psychomotor skills. Graduate nursing programs may focus on other types of assessment measures to establish progression such as successful completion of a predetermined number of clinical hours, documentation of accurate patient decisions related to advanced practice, and research activities.

Policies might regulate how many times a student may fail or withdraw from a course before being dismissed from the program. Some programs require students to complete all graduation requirements within a specific time period. Some programs use standardized tests to determine student progression between courses and between levels.

All decisions related to progression (and other nursing policies) should be based on data. Consider the following illustration that depicts evaluation with the goal of informing a decision on a progression policy. The faculty members at your school are considering student performance course examinations and grades earned related to their success on the NCLEX. Specific percentages earned for each of the nursing courses are tracked then correlated with the students' success on NCLEX. Faculty determined that 10 students from 100 graduating with the cohort failed NCLEX. The students who failed the NCLEX scored an average of 78 percent in each of the nursing courses. Faculty used this information to reset the passing percentage for nursing courses from 75 percent to 80 percent.

Graduation Policies

Graduation policies usually include stipulations that a student has successfully met program student learning outcomes, has completed all coursework with a minimum GPA, and has met all financial obligations to the school.

Graduation policies can also include high-stakes testing, requiring students to attain a certain score on a standardized examination to graduate from a program. Many schools have implemented high-stakes testing as part of their progression and graduation policies in an attempt to predict success on the NCLEX-RN (Nibert & Morrison, 2013). However, this practice is not without concern. Therefore, the NLN assembled a group of nursing and evaluation experts to study this practice. In February 2012, the NLN Board of Governors issued a document titled "The Fair Testing Imperative in Nursing Education." The text in Box 3.1 represents excerpts from this document. It is important for faculty to read the entire document prior to making decisions about using standardized examinations in their programs.

Another concern related to high-stakes testing and progression to graduation dependent on a score on a standardized exam is the assumption that can be made about the school's NCLEX pass rates. NCLEX pass rates are used by state boards of nursing and nursing accreditation agencies as a measure of a program's quality. However, if students are required to engage in prolonged remediation of nursing content for the purpose of passing a standardized exam before they are permitted to take NCLEX, the results are not representative of the nursing program but of the nursing program with additional study and remediation for the purpose of passing a standardized exam.

BOX 3.1 Excerpts from the NLN Fair Testing Imperative

Certainly, standardized test results are useful in various ways. They provide students with information about their knowledge compared with other students', using national norms; and they help faculty identify curricular strengths and weaknesses. But requiring a predetermined score for students to graduate and/or take the NCLEX in order to ensure that program pass rates remain at state board–prescribed levels is especially problematic for those who have successfully passed all other components of the nursing program. Students who cannot achieve the predetermined score may be forced to take the exit examination repeatedly until they achieve the score. They may fail the nursing course in which the test is a required component and endanger their standing in the nursing program. They may be denied their degrees or authorization to take the NCLEX. Cases like these can adversely affect the students and their families economically (i.e., while licensing is postponed, full salary potential is in jeopardy).

The Guidelines in Brief

1. Faculty have an ethical obligation to ensure that both tests and the decisions based on tests are valid; supported by solid evidence; consistent across courses; and fair to all test takers regardless of age, gender, disability, race, ethnicity, national origin, religion, sexual orientation, linguistic background, testing style and ability, or other personal characteristics.
2. Faculty have the responsibility to assess students' abilities and ensure that they are competent to practice nursing, while recognizing that current approaches to learning assessment are limited and imperfect.
3. Multiple sources of evidence are needed to evaluate basic nursing competence. Multiple approaches for assessment of knowledge and clinical abilities are particularly critical when high-stakes decisions (such as progression or graduation) are based on the assessment.
4. Tests and other evaluative measures should be used not only to evaluate student achievement, but, as importantly, to support student learning, improve teaching, and guide program improvements.
5. Comprehensive testing, administration, and evaluation information must be readily available to faculty before they administer, grade, and distribute results from, or write policies related to, the use of standardized tests. Faculty have the responsibility to review and incorporate these materials in communications to students about standardized testing and its consequences.

USE A VARIETY OF STRATEGIES TO ASSESS AND EVALUATE LEARNING ACROSS DOMAINS

Assessment and evaluation of learner achievement are designed to determine whether students have met intended objectives and outcomes and acquired the knowledge, skills, and abilities identified in the course, program, and curricula (Billings & Halstead, 2012). When selecting assessment and evaluation methods, the teacher chooses methods that best reflect the intended learning outcome. This ensures the assessment and evaluation strategies are valid because they are measuring what they are intended to measure.

Considerations when selecting assessment strategies include determining the setting for instruction and assessment (i.e., classroom or clinical site), as well as the domain of learning assessed. Bloom's classic taxonomy (1956) depicts the level of behavior at which competencies are demonstrated. Bloom addressed the domains

Table 3.1

Bloom's Taxonomy and Domains of Learning

Domain	Level (Highest to Lowest)
Cognitive	Creating Evaluating Analyzing Applying Understanding Remembering
Psychomotor	Naturalization Articulation Precision Manipulation Imitation
Affective	Internalizing the values Understanding the concept Conceptualizing and organizing Valuing Responding Receiving

of learning, including the cognitive, psychomotor, and affective domains. In the cognitive domain, the emphasis is on acquisition and use of knowledge, with levels ranging in a hierarchy from least to most complex (i.e., from remembering to creating) (Table 3.1). In the psychomotor domain, the focus is on performance of manual or physical skills, ranging from imitation to naturalization at the highest level. The affective domain incorporates emotions or feelings, and the concept ranges from receiving to internalizing values.

Teachers assessing learning in the cognitive domain commonly use objective tests and written assignments. The psychomotor domain provides a foundation for skills attainment in nursing and is most often assessed in the college skills laboratory, simulation laboratory, and clinical in a health care setting.

The affective domain, while sometimes more difficult to assess than the other two domains, is important in nursing education. Students often demonstrate learning in the affective domain through the use of creative writing, portfolios, and reflective journals. Clinical settings provide a venue where multiple domains may be assessed within a single experience. For example, a student caring for a patient who has an acute exacerbation of a severe illness may use critical thinking and decision-making skills to determine treatment (cognitive), perform a procedure (psychomotor), and demonstrate professionalism and empathy when working with the patient and the patient's family (affective).

CREATE ASSESSMENT INSTRUMENTS TO EVALUATE OUTCOMES

Teachers are responsible for developing assessment and evaluation strategies that yield meaningful data about student achievement and the effectiveness of the program. Assessment methods are designed to align with the lesson objectives and course for student learning outcomes (both content and level of thinking). For example, an objective in a beginning clinical nursing course laboratory assignment states, "The learner will accurately measure a patient's vital signs." An appropriate measure of performance is to have the student demonstrate assessment of vital signs on a partner or simulation manikin.

Methods must be valid and measure what students should have learned in the course. For example, if novice students are learning about the nursing process, a valid assessment method might include asking the student to describe the steps in the nursing process. Assessment strategies must also be reliable, or consistent, and produce similar results whenever the instrument is used. For example, all clinical sections of a course use standard measurement tools so all students are evaluated the same no matter who the clinical faculty might be. A consistent application of measurement in this instance supports interrater reliability.

USE ASSESSMENT INSTRUMENTS TO EVALUATE OUTCOMES; IMPLEMENT EVALUATION STRATEGIES APPROPRIATE TO THE LEARNER AND LEARNING OUTCOMES; ANALYZE AVAILABLE RESOURCES FOR LEARNER ASSESSMENT AND EVALUATION CRITERIA

Numerous instruments are available to evaluate learner attainment of outcomes. Whether assessing clinical or classroom performance, faculty should critically analyze available resources used in learner assessment and evaluation. Methods and tools should meet the following guidelines:

1. Instruments must be valid and reliable.
2. Assessment methods should align with lesson objectives and course student learning outcomes.
3. Lesson objectives must be measurable (Morrison, 2010).

A variety of assessment measures are used to determine attainment of outcomes. Multiple types of evaluation methods result in increased information and feedback, especially in formative evaluation, where it is possible to modify instruction as a result of assessment data.

Grading Rubrics

Grading rubrics assess student performance of subjective assignments using specific, measurable criteria. Typically, a grading rubric contains criteria that guide the student as to the level of expectations for the assignment and the teacher in grading the assignment. These criteria include a description of each area evaluated, the level of performance for each grading point, and an associated score. The most essential characteristic of a robust and meaningful rubric is that the data are measurable and directly connected to the student learning outcomes the assignment is designed to measure. Table 3.2 presents a sample rubric for a simple nursing diagnosis and plan of action assignment with a grading rubric.

Assessing Clinical Performance, Psychomotor Skills, and Affective Behaviors

Assessing clinical performance, psychomotor skills, and affective behaviors requires different methods of measurement than those used to evaluate classroom

Table 3.2

Sample Rubric for Nursing Diagnosis and Nursing Action Assignment

Criteria	Criteria Unmet 0 Points	Criteria Partially Met 1 Point	Criteria Met 2 Points
Correctly states 1 nursing diagnosis	Nursing diagnosis was not present	Nursing diagnosis was present but not correctly stated	Nursing diagnosis was present and correctly stated
Correctly states 3 nursing actions	Less than 3 nursing actions identified	Three nursing actions present, but not correctly stated	Three nursing actions were present and correctly stated

performance. Clinical evaluation is complex and affected by numerous factors, many that are outside the control of the faculty. Patient acuity, staffing levels, rapidly changing patient conditions, number and level of students, and clinical learning outcomes all impact straightforward evaluation of student performance in the clinical area. Subsequently, teachers use formative evaluation during the clinical course to provide ongoing feedback throughout the clinical day and to adjust to student learning needs.

Clinical evaluation instruments are developed to provide specific, measurable criteria consistent with course student learning outcomes (Bonnel, 2012). According to Bonnel, primary strategies for evaluating clinical practice include observation, oral communication, written communication, simulation, and self-evaluation. Observation allows the teacher to see student performance and may support the use of checklists and anecdotal notes to support assessment. Grading rubrics are commonly used to evaluate clinical performance, depicting a range from satisfactory to unsatisfactory or points on a numerical scale to rate student achievement.

In the era of high-fidelity clinical simulators, scenarios and case studies have become a universal method for both practice and evaluation. Measurement of cognitive, affective, and psychomotor behaviors, ranging from simple to complex, may be accomplished with the use of clinical simulation. Case studies and patient scenarios can provide realistic environments for care, enhanced by multimedia equipment that yields immediate feedback, allows for unlimited practice in a safe environment, and enables self-evaluation.

Assessing affective behaviors may be challenging, but a number of methods have been used in nursing education for this purpose. Student self-reflection and self-evaluation are supported by the use of reflective journals and clinical logs. Clinical portfolios are used as a means to collect a collage of artifacts that reflect learning and achievement over time. There are many ways to develop a clinical portfolio. Faculty should become familiar with the types of portfolios used and select the one that best meets the desired outcome.

Student self-assessment is an important aspect of most nursing programs and assessment in a variety of educational settings including the classroom, clinical, and nursing laboratories. Reflection upon a learning experience is an affective behavior that allows students to consider their own performance based on expected assignment learning outcomes. Reflective journals and portfolios support self-assessment and may be used to demonstrate higher-level and abstract thinking.

Classroom Assessment

Classroom assessment is accomplished through a variety of strategies used to assess student achievement of student learning outcomes. Assignments such as papers, debates, audio and video recordings, presentations, group projects, journals, simulation and gaming, portfolios, reflection, role play, service learning, and concept mapping are all used to assess and evaluate student learning.

Developing Valid and Reliable Tests

In *The Scope of Practice for Academic Nurse Educators,* the NLN (2012b) states that teaching, learning, and evaluation strategies are evidence-based. Creating valid and reliable tests and using standard metrics to examine outcomes of testing provide the nurse educator with evidence of dependable measures that yield a high level of confidence in the results. Faculty must have confidence that the evaluation methods provide the most accurate measure of the students' achievement of the student learning outcomes. An important task of faculty is to eliminate irrelevant variance from these measures. That is, the results obtained from the instruments used to evaluate student learning are not influenced by any factors other than the student's learning. Eliminating all irrelevant variance is impossible, but should be the goal when developing and using evaluation instruments.

Constructing valid and reliable tests requires skill, practice, and time. When planning to test students, the teacher first determines the purpose of the testing. If the test is administered prior to instruction, it may reflect readiness or placement. When administered during instruction, it serves as a formative evaluation of learning. When administered at the conclusion of the instruction, the test serves as summative evaluation of learning and may provide information to determine progression and grading (Twigg, 2012). Numerous tools assist the teacher in test development including a test blueprint, test storage and retrieval databases, and test analysis software.

Test Blueprints

Development of a test blueprint, a map that connects content and outcomes to the test items, is one method used to address content validity of an exam. Faculty develop a test blueprint prior to creating an exam and include the course or unit outcome or content, the expected cognitive level (Bloom's taxonomy), the total number of desired test items, and the weight or percentage of the exam allotted to each area. In testing prelicensure nursing students, categories may be added that include the NCLEX-RN test plan and steps in the nursing process (Morrison, 2010). An additional consideration is the level of difficulty of items, which should correlate with the learning level of the students and the expected mastery level of the content. Numerous examples of tables and spreadsheets, including some that are computer generated, are available for nurse educators to use when developing a test blueprint. Table 3.3 depicts a sample test blueprint, relating content areas to the nursing process, assigning weight to each area, and classifying according to cognitive level. This blueprint is a summative type of test blueprint. Another type of blueprint tracks each test item of specific importance to the teacher. Table 3.4 provides an example of a test blueprint that demonstrates congruency among the test item, lesson objective, and course student learning outcomes. This type of test blueprint is preferred because it demonstrates a higher level of specificity for the validity of the test items.

Table 3.3

Sample Test Blueprint Using Nursing Process Content Areas on a
100-Item Exam

Outcome/Content Area	Percentage of Exam in Content Area	Cognitive Level: Knowledge	Cognitive Level: Comprehension	Cognitive Level: Application
Assessment	25%	8	7	9
Diagnosis	20%	6	6	8
Planning	15%	4	4	7
Intervention	15%	5	5	7
Evaluation	25%	7	8	9
Total	100%	30	30	40

Table 3.4

Test Blueprint Aligning Test Items to the Lesson Objective and Course
Student Learning Outcome

Question	Lesson Objective	Course Student Learning Outcome	Step in the Nursing Process	Other Nursing Situation	NCLEX Category	Cognitive Level	Difficulty Level of Key	Item Discrimination of Key
1								
2								
3								
4								
5								
6								
7								
8								
9								
10								
11								
12								

When selecting the number of test items, the teacher takes into account a number of considerations, including the level of the student and the time available for testing. Although test reliability may increase with the number of test items, there may be time limitations. A general guideline is to allow approximately 1 minute per each multiple-choice test item. Items that require higher-level thinking may require more time to answer than those that test a lower level of thinking.

Test Construction and Item Writing

Objective tests assess understanding of content and the ability to think at the knowledge, comprehension, application, and analysis levels. Test items are designed to measure competency or mastery of a subject. Objective-style examinations permit testing a number of students at one time and may be scored rapidly, often with the use of computerized scoring equipment that offers item analysis. Disadvantages of objective testing include the difficulty in writing items that examine critical thinking skills, as well as the time needed to develop valid, reliable tests.

Developing and selecting the format for test items is time-consuming and requires skill and practice. Item format is determined by considering which of the multiple types of formats most directly measures the intended learning outcome (Twigg, 2012). The most common item formats include multiple choice, true or false, matching, short answer, fill in the blank, and ordered response. A form of multiple choice, labeled multiple response, includes several correct responses. The NCLEX-RN uses alternative format questions, including fill in the blank, multiple response, drag and drop, ordered response, picture or graphic, and audio questions.

Regardless of the format selected, exams should include high-level, critical thinking test items. Morrison, Nibert, and Flick (2006) identified four criteria for developing critical thinking test items: (a) include rationales; (b) are at the application or higher cognitive level; (c) require a high level of discrimination to select the correct answer from plausible distracters; and (d) require multilogical thinking, also known as sequential reasoning, where more than one step in the thinking process is required to answer a question.

Multiple-choice test items typically include the question, referred to as the stem, and a set of responses, with the correct response referred to as the key and the incorrect responses distracters. When writing the stem, the teacher should include clear, unbiased language and avoid giving overt clues to the correct answer. Responses should be plausible and at approximately the same length and level of complexity. All items should be referenced in the test blueprint and should be checked for accuracy.

ANALYZE ASSESSMENT AND EVALUATION DATA

Collecting data is the first step of the assessment and evaluation process, but careful analysis of the data is critical to performing evidence-based assessment. Teachers use multiple means of measuring student performance, then accurately interpret the data to produce an indicator of student learning that is reliable. Understanding test results may be confusing and requires knowledge of some basic concepts as well as experience to gain skill and confidence.

Analyzing Test Results

One of the most important aspects of testing is completion of a statistical analysis. The purpose of completing a statistical analysis on test items is to ensure exams are effectively evaluating student learning. The three measures most important in test analysis are (a) difficulty level of each of the test items contained on the exam, (b) item discrimination for the key and all distracters, and (c) the exam's reliability (Morrison et al., 2006).

Most nursing programs rely on the use of test scoring software, such as Scan-Tron®, ParSYSTEM®, and LXR Test®, to assist with test development, storage, blue printing, and analysis. With the ease of using these systems, much of the manual calculation of test item statistics is eliminated. It is, however, extremely important for teachers to understand the reports generated by the testing software. When considering such a system, teachers should explore a number of factors, including cost of the product, ease of use and available training, depth and accuracy of results, and ongoing support from the distributor.

Difficulty Level

When evaluating exam results, the teacher first considers if the examination was too difficult or too easy. Exam difficulty may be determined through reviewing the mean, median, and mode, where the mean is the average of the group scores on an exam, the median is the halfway point where one-half of the students scored above this number and one-half scored below, and the mode is the most frequently obtained score (Morrison, 2010). To effectively measure different levels of student learning, exams include items of varying levels of difficulty. Item difficulty (p value), also called the difficulty level, difficulty factor, or difficulty index, measures the percentage of students who answered a test item correctly. The range would be reported, for example, as 0.00 to 1.00. For example, a difficulty factor of 0.76 means that 76 percent of the students answered an item correctly. According to Morrison (2010), an acceptable level of difficulty is 30 to 90 percent.

Item Discrimination

The second area to consider when evaluating test results is whether the item discriminated between those students who knew the content and those who did not, which is determined by the grade earned on that exam. For each item, this statistic reflects how those students who scored highest on the exam answered that item. The item discrimination factor compares the number of students who answered the item correctly based on their overall score on the exam with those who did not score as well. It is assumed that a higher number of high-scoring students should have answered the item correctly than low-scoring students.

An effective exam question will discriminate between the students who have learned at a higher level and those individuals scoring at a lower level. According to Morrison (2010), item discrimination is the best indicator of the quality of a test item because it shows the item's ability to differentiate between high-scoring and low-scoring students. For example, if students with high test scores answer an item correctly, and students with low overall test scores answer the item incorrectly, the item is said to discriminate, or differentiate, between those who do and those who do not know the material. If, however, a larger number of low-scoring students on the exam more often answered the question correctly than high-scoring students, the question is not reliable in differentiating between those who know and those who do not know the material.

Two commonly used methods for item discrimination include the item discrimination ratio (IDR) (sometimes called the *discrimination index*) and the point biserial correlation coefficient (PBCC) (Morrison, 2010). Although the IDR is more easily calculated, the PBCC is considered the more robust measurement of item discrimination.

The IDR assesses high-scoring and low-scoring student responses to test items. An acceptable level for the IDR is 25 percent. The IDR is calculated by considering the top 27 percent and bottom 27 percent of the student scores as follows:

IDR = a – b
a = response frequency (percentage) of the top 27 percent of students on an item
b = response frequency (percentage) of the lowest 27 percent of students on an item

For example, if 75 percent of the top-scoring students answered an item correctly, and 50 percent of the lowest-scoring students answered an item correctly, the IDR is 25 percent (i.e., IDR = 75 percent – 50 percent = 25 percent). The most accurate measure of an item's level of discrimination is its PBCC. For enterprising faculty, Morrison (2010, p. 22) offers a formula for calculating the PBCC. Test analysis software, however, is now available to assist the teacher in quickly determining the PBCC, so calculating this manually is rare. Instead, it is more important to be able to interpret analysis reports correctly than to spend time with manual calculations.

As mentioned, an understanding of the significance of the PBCC score is critical. The PBCC ranges from –1.00 to 1.00, where a positive point biserial indicates that high-scoring students answered a test item correctly more frequently than low-scoring students, and a negative point biserial indicates low-scoring students answered a test item correctly more frequently than high-scoring students. The higher the PBCC, the better the item discriminates between low and high achievers on an examination (McDonald, 2007). According to McDonald, a PBCC above 0.20 defines a highly discriminating item on an exam, adding that items with a PBCC of lower than 0.20 should be revised. A zero PBCC indicates that students who did well and those who did poorly on the exam answered the item correctly with equal frequency. Items that are very easy or very difficult will have a low discrimination level.

In addition to analyzing overall PBCC for each test item, the teacher also critically examines each item's details (i.e., the difficulty [p value] and PBCC of the distracters for each test item). For example, consider Table 3.5 for examples of results of two test items.

Item 1 represents a statistically stable question, where the item difficulty of 0.69 and the PBCC of 0.42 reflect the item discriminated well between high-scoring and low-scoring students. The negative PBCC on each of the incorrect items indicates low-scoring students selected the incorrect items more frequently than the high-scoring students. A different picture is reflected in item 2. Although the difficulty level of 0.75

Table 3.5

Interpreting Individual Item Results

Item Number	Difficulty (p Value)	Overall Item PBCC	Option	Response Proportion	PBCC
1	0.69	0.42	A	0.03	–0.46
			B	0.23	–0.30
			C	0.69	0.42
			D	0.05	–0.28
2	0.75	0.09	A	0.75	0.09
			B	0.08	–0.28
			C	0.11	0.08
			D	0.06	–0.26

is sufficient, the correct response is shown to be a poor discriminator with a PBCC of 0.09, with distracter C also having a positive PBCC. The teacher would consider accepting answer C in this case or modifying the item before using it again. For both items all distracters were selected by students taking the exam. This is a positive finding. If there are distracters that no students chose, then the distracter is not distracting the uninformed student and is not functioning as a distracter. If there are four options and no students choose one of the options because it is obviously wrong, students now have a one in three chance of correctly guessing the answer rather than a one in four chance. This makes the item less reliable if the chance for guessing the correct answer is increased. Therefore, distracters that are not selected by any students should be rewritten or eliminated. These distracters are causing the student to spend time reading them but are not functioning for the purpose for which they were intended.

Reliability

Finally, when examining test results, the teacher asks, "What was the reliability of the exam?" Reliability refers to the consistency of test results; it is the degree to which test scores are free from measurement error (Morrison, 2010). There are a number of measures of reliability, including test-retest, parallel form, and internal consistency.

Test-retest reliability requires administering the identical test to the same individual on a second occasion, and then determining the correlation between the scores. In parallel-form reliability, two different forms of the test are administered to the same person, with the results of the two tests then being correlated. Both of these methods are unfeasible for most classroom teachers due to time constraints and difficulty in creating equivalent forms of a test.

When considering internal consistency and reliability, the Kuder-Richardson (KR-20) is commonly used to measure interitem consistency (Morrison, 2010). Like the PBCC, the range of the KR-20 will fall between –1.0 and 1.0, where a reliability coefficient of 1.0 indicates perfect reliability, and a reliability coefficient of 0.0 indicates the test lacks reliability. Morrison notes it is rare to see a negative KR-20, as this would mean that many of the test items are being answered correctly by low-scoring students instead of high-scoring students. A KR-20 score of 0.60 is acceptable for teacher-made nursing examinations. *Kuder- Richardson*

Using Standardized Exams

Many schools of nursing employ the use of commercially available tests to supplement faculty-developed exams. Standardized tests have become a common means of demonstrating evaluation of programs and are frequently found on a nursing program's systematic evaluation plan. When selecting these exams, faculty carefully consider a number of variables, including detailed information about content and how the content included on the examination was determined, data on validity and reliability, and the level of competence tested. Faculty often discuss the attributes of various commercial exams with other users and find that anecdotal information about exams, as well as the support offered by the test agency, will influence purchasing decisions. The reader is referred to the NLN's position statement on the fair use of standardized examinations, as previously discussed.

ADVISE LEARNERS REGARDING ASSESSMENT AND EVALUATION CRITERIA

Faculty members are responsible for apprising students of the criteria on which they will be evaluated. In some instances this is provided through academic bulletins or handbooks that outline formal policies related to course expectations, academic progression, standardized testing, and clinical expectations. Course syllabi should clearly define these expectations, providing clear descriptions and expectations of assignments and evaluation methods.

Providing learners with test blueprints, detailed assignment grading rubrics, and clearly delineated expectations supports both the student and the faculty conducting the assessment. If clinical evaluation is part of the course, students are provided objective, measurable performance criteria to guide their behavior.

Providing straightforward communication of all expectations to students supports positive outcomes and helps avoid confusion and misunderstanding. Transparency regarding assessment and evaluation criteria also supports the delivery of growth-producing feedback to students.

PROVIDE TIMELY, CONSTRUCTIVE, AND THOUGHTFUL FEEDBACK TO LEARNERS

Formative evaluation, as previously mentioned, is used to provide feedback to support learning. When providing student feedback, the teacher considers a number of criteria. Feedback should be timely, specific, and constructive. Effective feedback is given as close to the time of assessment as possible, allowing students to modify their behavior and respond to a learning experience. Feedback should provide specific information for the student to use to improve performance. Feedback addresses both strengths and areas for development as well as what steps to take to achieve expected outcomes. Constructive feedback focuses on specific ways to improve performance.

In addition to written assignments and examinations, nursing faculty may use midterm and/or end-of-term conferences to discuss performance (DeYoung, 2009). The content discussed about clinical performance should be concrete and specific. It is important to focus on specific behaviors, including what is right, what is wrong, why it is wrong, and how the behavior may be corrected. For example, it would be better to tell a student, "In performing the patient's dressing change, you did not follow sterile technique. You contaminated the site with your sleeve, and your hair was in the sterile field," rather than, "You need to improve your sterile technique." When students perform poorly or demonstrate unsafe behaviors in the clinical area, the teacher should immediately meet with the student to discuss the performance and create a plan for improvement. For unsafe behaviors, close supervision is required until the faculty evaluates the student as providing safe patient care.

SUMMARY

Assessment and evaluation data inform decisions about courses, programs, curriculum, and educational standards and policies. Nurse educators are accountable for understanding and using evidence-based assessment and evaluation methods in classroom and clinical settings. A variety of evaluation strategies should be used to measure all domains of learning. Many strategies support assessment and evaluation of learner outcomes across learning domains.

Practice Test Questions

1. Which best represents the purpose of a summative clinical evaluation tool?
  A. Determination of the relative effect of education on the students' weekly clinical performance
  B. Assessment of students' acquisition of knowledge and skills during a particular clinical experience
  C. Determination that learning occurred and behavioral objectives were met during the semester
  D. Assessment of all activities associated with students' clinical experience over the duration of the program

2. Which best describes a criterion-referenced assessment activity?
  A. Interpretation of data in terms of a norm or group
  B. Evaluation of mastery of specified outcomes
  C. Use of information for predictive purpose
  D. Comparison of data between groups

3. The nursing instructor decides to grade an exam on a curve. This is an example of which of the following?
  A. Criterion referencing
  B. Norm referencing
  C. Summative evaluation
  D. Formative evaluation

4. A nursing course is taught by three nurse educators who share responsibility for classroom content, laboratory time, and clinical experiences. When evaluating students in this course, what must the faculty do to ensure that students are receiving fair grades?
  A. Weekly meetings of the faculty members to evaluate students
  B. All students are evaluated by the same faculty member
  C. Faculty members establish interrater reliability for the course evaluation strategies
  D. Students are graded solely on a final exam prepared by all faculty in the course

Exam Item	Difficulty Factor	Item Discrimination (Point Biserial Correlation Coefficient)	Reliability (KR-20)
1	26%	0.39	0.80
2	32%	0.68	0.76

5. In the above item analysis, which of the following statements is correct?
  A. The reliability of the items is poor.
  B. In item 2, the lower scoring students answered the question correctly.
  C. The difficulty factor of both items is within an acceptable range.
  D. The item discrimination (point biserial correlation coefficient) indicates that the item discriminates well between low-scoring and high-scoring students.

(continued on page 66)

Individual Item Statistics					
Item Number	**Difficulty (*p* Value)**	**Overall Item PBCC**	**Option**	**Response Proportion**	**PBCC**
1	0.75	0.09	A	0.75	0.09
			B	0.08	−0.28
			C	0.11	0.08
			D	0.06	−0.26

6. In the above item analysis, which of the following statements is correct?
   A. Seventy-five percent of the students answered the question correctly.
   B. More high-scoring students selected answer B than low-scoring students.
   C. More low-scoring students selected A than high-scoring students.
   D. This is a highly discriminating item.

7. The novice nurse educator is reviewing item analysis results from a recent examination. She demonstrates that she understands the purpose of item analysis when she states:
   A. "I am looking for items that may be too difficult, too easy, or had two correct answers."
   B. "I want to find ways to give the students extra points."
   C. "I want to have proof so that the students can't argue with the results."
   D. "The results will show me how to make the test easier next time."

8. The teacher develops the following question:
   Contact precautions should be used for a client who has a disease transmitted by:
   a. Tiny airborne droplet nuclei
   b. Blood-borne pathogens
   c. Inhaling large particle droplets
   d. Touching a contaminated object

   Which Bloom's taxonomy level is being tested in the above item?
   A. Knowledge
   B. Comprehension
   C. Application
   D. Analysis

9. The nursing instructor is preparing new items for an examination on neurological assessment for the health assessment course. Which of these stems measure learning at the analysis level?
   A. Which cranial nerve is being tested by observing the cardinal positions of gaze?
   B. The nurse observes that the patient's tongue deviates to one side and there is right-sided hemiplegia. What other neurological tests can the nurse include in the assessment to validate a diagnosis of cerebrovascular accident?
   C. The nurse is initiating a care plan for a patient just admitted with Parkinson's disease and aspiration pneumonia. Which of these nursing diagnoses should take priority?
   D. Which of these statements by the mother of a child recently diagnosed with Duchenne's dystrophy suggests the need for further teaching?

References

Billings, D. M., & Halstead, J. A. (Eds.). (2012). *Teaching in nursing: A guide for faculty.* (4th ed.). St. Louis: Elsevier.

Bloom, B. S. (1956). *Taxonomy of educational objectives: The classification of educational goals.* New York: Longman.

Bonnel, W. (2012). Clinical performance evaluation. In D. M. Billings & J. A. Halstead (Eds.), *Teaching in nursing: A guide for faculty* (4th ed., pp. 485–502). St. Louis: Elsevier.

DeYoung, S. (2009). *Teaching strategies for nurse educators* (2nd ed.). Upper Saddle River, NJ: Prentice-Hall Health.

Frank, B. (2010). No nursing student left untested: The role of standardized testing within nursing curricula. In L. Caputi (Ed.), *Teaching nursing: The art and science* (2nd ed., Vol. 3, pp. 28–44). Glen Ellyn, IL: College of DuPage Press.

McDonald, M. (2007). *The nurse educator's guide to assessing learning outcomes* (2nd ed.). Sudbury, MA: Jones and Bartlett.

Morrison, S. (2010). Test construction and item writing. In L. Caputi (Ed.), *Teaching nursing: The art and science* (2nd ed., Vol. 3, pp. 2–27). Glen Ellyn, IL: College of DuPage Press.

Morrison, S., Nibert, A., & Flick, J. (2006). *Critical thinking and test item writing* (2nd ed.). Houston, TX: Health Education Systems.

National League for Nursing (NLN). (2012a, February). The fair testing imperative in nursing education. Retrieved from http://www.nln.org/aboutnln/livingdocuments/pdf/nlnvision_4.pdf

National League for Nursing (NLN). (2012b). *The scope of practice for academic nurse educators.* Philadelphia: Lippincott Williams & Wilkins.

Nibert, A., & Morrison, S. (2013). HESI testing: A history of evidence-based research. *Journal of Professional Nursing, 29*(25), S2–S4.

Oermann, M., & Gaberson, K. (2009). *Evaluation and testing in nursing education* (3rd ed.). New York: Springer.

Twigg, P. (2012). Developing and using classroom tests. In D. M. Billings & J. A. Halstead (Eds.), *Teaching in nursing: A guide for faculty* (4th ed., pp. 464–484). St. Louis: Elsevier.

Participate in Curriculum Design and Evaluation of Program Outcomes

Linda Caputi, EdD, RN, CNE, ANEF

The CNE Test Plan Lists the Following for the Area of Participate in Curriculum Design and Evaluation of Program Outcomes:

4. Participate in Curriculum Design and Evaluation of Program Outcomes

- **A.** Demonstrate knowledge of curriculum development including:
  - **1.** identifying program outcomes
  - **2.** developing competency statements
  - **3.** writing course objectives
  - **4.** selecting appropriate learning activities
  - **5.** selecting appropriate clinical experiences
  - **6.** selecting appropriate evaluation strategies
- **B.** Actively participate in the design of the curriculum to reflect:
  - **1.** institutional philosophy and mission
  - **2.** current nursing and health care trends
  - **3.** community and societal needs
  - **4.** nursing principles, standards, theory, and research
  - **5.** educational principles, theory, and research
  - **6.** use of technology
- **C.** Lead the development of curriculum design
- **D.** Lead the development of course design
- **E.** Analyze results of program evaluation
- **F.** Revise the curriculum based on evaluation of:
  - **1.** program outcomes
  - **2.** learner needs
  - **3.** societal and health care trends
  - **4.** stakeholder feedback (e.g., from learners, agency personnel, accrediting agencies, advisory boards)
- **G.** Implement curricular revisions using appropriate change theories and strategies
- **H.** Collaborate with community and clinical partners to support educational goals
- **I.** Design program assessment plans that promote continuous quality improvement
- **J.** Implement the program assessment plan
- **K.** Evaluate the program assessment plan

The task statements noted in the detailed Certified Nurse Educator test blueprint for Competency 4 reflect the nurse educator's role in the important function of developing, implementing, and evaluating the nursing program curriculum. The word *curriculum* can be defined in a number of ways. Faculty working together in a school of nursing should all use the same definition of the word *curriculum* as well as an understanding of what curriculum revision entails. This chapter covers the design, development, and evaluation of a curriculum and addresses the specific responsibilities of faculty as active participants in curriculum design and evaluation of program outcomes.

DEMONSTRATE KNOWLEDGE OF CURRICULUM DEVELOPMENT; ACTIVELY PARTICIPATE IN THE DESIGN OF THE CURRICULUM

Developing a curriculum is an organized, systematic process. The overall intent of a curriculum is to develop a program plan of study that results in graduates exhibiting characteristics reflective of what they have learned in the nursing program. This requires determining the desired characteristics students will display upon successful completion of all coursework in the program. These characteristics are known as learning outcomes or student learning outcomes (SLOs). Program SLOs are broad statements. Most nursing programs write from six to nine program SLOs. Because these SLOs are the intended outcomes of the program of study, they must be measured to ensure they are achieved. Therefore, the beginning point is to write measurable SLOs as the end product of the program. However, because program SLOs are broad statements, they can be difficult to measure. Competencies for each program SLO provide more detailed behaviors for each SLO; these competencies are measurable. The American Nurses Association defined a competency as "an expected level of performance that integrates knowledge, skills, abilities, and judgment" (ANA, 2008, p. 3). The following is an example program SLO with related competency statements:

Example program SLO: Participate in quality improvement processes to improve patient care.
Example competencies for the SLO:

1. Apply quality improvement processes to effectively implement patient safety initiatives and monitor performance measures, including nursing-sensitive indicators.
2. Analyze information gathered using quality improvement metrics to identify changes for improved patient outcomes.
3. Identify gaps between local and best practice and provide recommendations for closing the gaps.
4. Participate in analyzing errors and identifying system improvements.

The specific competencies provide measurable behaviors to determine if the student has met the program SLO of "Participate in quality improvement processes to improve patient care."

The Basis for Program SLOs

If writing the program SLOs is the first step in development of a curriculum, the question is What is the basis for these program SLOs? There are a number of important entities faculty must consider when writing program SLOs (Caputi, 2010):

1. *The institutional philosophy, mission, and learning outcomes.* Nursing programs generally reside within a larger institutional setting. The institution typically presents learners with a philosophy or mission that provides information about the focus of that institution and why it exists. These are often expressed as the institution's value statements, which provide overall direction for the philosophy or

mission of the nursing program. The institution may also have general educational learning outcomes that all students graduating from that institution will achieve. The nursing program SLOs ensure those general educational learning outcomes are met as an expression of the nursing program SLOs. For example, if an institutional level educational outcome is "Engage in critical thinking," a nursing program SLO might be, "Engage in clinical reasoning to provide quality patient care." Therefore, the nursing program SLO supports the institutional-level educational learning outcome.

2. *Regulatory requirements.* Regulatory requirements refer to the state board of nursing's requirements for the nursing program. There are a wide range of requirements among state boards of nursing. Some boards of nursing are very detailed in the curriculum requirements such as those presented by the Texas State Board of Nursing's Differentiated Essential Competencies. Other boards of nursing are not as detailed in their expectations related to curriculum and provide general guidelines to which nursing schools must comply.

3. *Accreditation agencies.* Both the Accreditation Commission for Education in Nursing, Inc. (ACEN, 2013) and the Commission on Collegiate Nursing Education (CCNE, 2013) provide standards related to curriculum. For example, ACEN's Standard 4, the curriculum standard, has a number of criteria with specific expectations. Two examples are (a) the curriculum incorporates established professional standards, guidelines, and competencies and has clearly articulated student learning outcomes and program outcomes consistent with contemporary practice, and (b) the student learning outcomes are used to organize the curriculum, guide the delivery of instruction, direct learning activities, and evaluate student progress. Accredited programs must ensure their curricula meet these accreditation requirements.

4. *Licensing and certification exam requirements.* Another major influence on the nursing curriculum are the national exams graduates must pass to practice. Prelicensure curricula should include coverage of the National Council Licensure Examination for Registered Nurses for Practical Nurses and Registered Nurses (NCLEX-PN® and NCLEX-RN®) test plan. Graduate programs should include coverage of the expectations of certification examinations required for advanced practice licensure. The content on the test plans as well as the cognitive level at which the exams are written are equally important.

5. *Current nursing and health care trends and community and societal needs.* Nursing faculty must ensure the program curriculum addresses current nursing and health care trends and needs as well as specific community and societal needs, such as addressing diversity or specific regional and societal needs in communities in which the graduates will practice. A broad, current knowledge base related to patient and community needs is an important element for a curriculum to address. This includes gathering information from the program's stakeholders such as the agencies that employ the school's graduates, understanding the needs of the community the schools serve, and incorporating current trends in health care including improving patient outcomes. The goal in developing curriculum is to ensure that it addresses the current health care environment, which requires ongoing efforts by faculty to remain current in nursing practice. It requires a knowledge of professional standards including nursing principles, standards of care, theory, and research with implementation of each in the nursing program at the appropriate level for the type of nursing program. This means faculty must make deliberate decisions about how these professional standards are taught depending on the type of program (licensed practical nurse, associate

degree in nursing, diploma, bachelor of nursing science, master's of science in nursing, doctor of nursing practice, or other doctoral level programs). The differentiated outcomes and competencies developed by the National League for Nursing (NLN, 2010) are useful when making these decisions.

As indicated by this discussion, curriculum is no longer solely based on a nursing theorist or other established theoretical framework. Curriculum building is based on current nursing practice, the needs of the patients in the health care system, and a number of influencing initiatives. Although becoming outdated, some faculty may use the terms *organizing framework* or *theoretical framework* to represent the basis on which the curriculum is structured. Developing a curriculum that meets current health care needs requires faculty to maintain currency in both the practice and academic environments to ensure the curriculum does not become stagnant and outdated. The term *outdated* in a rapidly changing health care environment means a much shorter shelf life for curriculum (Halstead, 2007). A curriculum that has not been updated in five years may have become outdated. Curriculum revision is an ongoing process. Once a curriculum has been developed based on current initiatives, as previously noted, a yearly review and revision based on the results of evaluation of SLOs and other program evaluation metrics as well as recent initiatives in nursing and health care over that current year are required.

Faculty must be well versed in the entities that oversee or guide curriculum to ensure compliance during the process of developing and implementing the curriculum. Being cognizant of these influences is important to ensure the curriculum not only provides the means for students to achieve the student learning outcomes, but also for the program to achieve program outcomes. SLOs are what individual students will achieve; program outcomes are what a group or cohort of students will achieve as a result of completing the nursing program. Program outcomes include measures such as NCLEX pass rates, certification exam pass rates, employer satisfaction with graduates' ability to engage in current nursing practice, graduate satisfaction with the nursing program in preparing them to engage in current nursing practice, retention rate, and employment rate. Development of current, evidence-based SLOs that provide the educational basis for students to perform individually and as a group as measured by achievement of program SLOs and competencies and positive results on program outcomes is the hallmark of an excellent curriculum.

LEAD THE DEVELOPMENT OF CURRICULUM AND COURSE DESIGN

Once the program SLOs and competencies have been written, faculty must develop the courses. Content is one of the two major focuses of the curriculum. The other focus is how to use the content. Initially, faculty determine what content will be taught in the program, then level the content throughout the nursing courses. However, content alone is insufficient. Students must know how to use the content, what content to use, and how to apply the content when engaging in clinical reasoning for the purpose of providing safe, quality, evidence-based, patient-centered care. Therefore, both content and thinking are leveled as students advance through the nursing courses. Bloom's taxonomy is used to demonstrate increasing levels of competency when writing course SLOs and competencies (Anderson et al. 2001).

Because the purpose of the curriculum is to ensure students are able to achieve the program SLOs and competencies, nursing courses are built so they apply the program SLOs and competencies into each course. This provides evidence that each course is structured to culminate in the program's SLOs and competencies.

Faculty determine the sequencing of courses, building on content and thinking expectations. This is often a challenge for faculty as they determine the arrangement of content within courses and the arrangement of the course within the curriculum. Faculty should apply a specific plan for making these decisions. A variety of curriculum models can be used. For example, many programs still use the traditional body systems approach to arranging content. Within this traditional approach, content is arranged according to specialty practice areas such as pediatrics, mental health, care of adults, and so forth. Other programs are transitioning to a concept-based curriculum. A concept-based curriculum arranges content around concepts important to the practice of nursing and presents those concepts "across environmental settings, the life span, and the health-illness continuum" (Giddens & Brady, 2007, p. 67). A truly concept-based curriculum can be one solution to content saturation, which has plagued nursing curricula for decades and is growing increasingly worse with the rapid expansion of knowledge.

Learning Activities, Clinical Experiences, and Evaluation Strategies

Once course content has been structured and course SLOs and competencies have been developed, faculty plan the implementation of the curriculum. Questions addressed in this stage include: (a) What content and thinking skills will be taught? (b) How will the content and thinking skills be taught? (c) How will the content and thinking be applied in laboratory experiences such as the clinical, skills lab, and simulation lab? (d) How will achievement of course SLOs be evaluated? These questions are best answered using a tool such as a lesson plan. A lesson plan demonstrates a direct line of congruency among the course SLOs and competencies, the unit lesson objectives, the teaching-learning strategies used to deliver the lesson, and the evaluation strategies. Table 4.1 provides an example lesson plan.

The lesson plan provides evidence of the linkage of what happens in the classroom to the course SLOs and competencies, which are directly reflective of the program SLOs and competencies. Oftentimes faculty have difficulty demonstrating this connection. The lesson plan provides this evidence. The specific unit objectives provide details about what is taught, which is a major decision for many faculty because most nursing programs tend to teach more content than is realistic for students to process. Students who are overloaded with content tend to resort to rote memorization of information rather than engaging in active learning and higher level processing. Faculty must resist the temptation to teach volumes of information and to continually add content as nursing knowledge grows. There is no evidence for the underlying assumption that as long as content is "covered," thinking follows; that is, covering content does not in itself promote critical thinking and clinical reasoning (Giddens & Brady, 2007; Ironside, 2004). A process for cutting content that provides general guidelines for what is or is not taught is critical to developing a successful curriculum. For example, rather than covering all diseases presented under a particular topic (such as the respiratory system or the concept of oxygenation), faculty can develop a process for deciding the top five respiratory diseases currently treated in the United States and then focus on those five. Other guidelines might relate to any additional diseases specific to the region in which the school is located and the top three medications used to treat each of the five identified diseases.

Table 4.1

Sample Lesson Plan

Course SLO	Competency	Unit Objectives	Teaching-Learning Strategies	Evaluation Methods
1. Demonstrate critical thinking and clinical reasoning to make patient-centered care decisions when caring for child-bearing families and children.	1.1 Use critical thinking/clinical reasoning to make clinical judgments and care management decisions for the childbearing family and children to ensure accurate and safe care in all nursing actions.	**Classroom/Lab:** • Use critical thinking/clinical reasoning when making clinical judgments and management decisions to ensure accurate and safe care.	**Classroom:** • Unfolding case study, small group work assignments, then discussion to develop a concept map. • Practice items using clickers. **Clinical:** • Concept map to demonstrate links related to assessment data and nursing care with tie to clinical judgment and management decisions. • Concept map to include plans for safe care.	**Classroom:** • Unit exam: Three application-level questions included on test blueprint. **Clinical:** • Clinical evaluation tool to include competency. • Concept map with grading rubric.
	1.2 Use critical thinking/clinical reasoning when implementing all steps of the nursing process while integrating best available evidence.	**Classroom/Lab:** • Use critical thinking/clinical reasoning to plan care using the nursing process. • Identify sources of information for best available evidence for the childbearing family and children.	**Classroom:** • Review of reliable websites for evidence-based nursing practice. • Small group work continuing the development of the concept map. • Group discussion of completed map. **Clinical:** • Concept map to include sources of best available evidence used to plan care.	**Classroom:** • Unit exam: Two analysis-level questions included on test blueprint. **Clinical:** • Clinical evaluation tool to include competency. • Concept map with grading rubric.
	1.3 Anticipate common risks associated with the childbearing family and stable pediatric patients, and predict and manage potential complications.	**Classroom/Lab:** • Discuss types of patient data to use when planning care to decrease risks and predict and manage potential complications for the childbearing family and children.	**Classroom:** • Discuss use of informatics for data mining related to common complications and quality improvement metrics. • Small group work circling assessment data that indicate potential risks. • Group to discuss nursing interventions to prevent/manage potential complications. • Group discussion of completed map. **Clinical:** • Include on concept map specific patient data linked to potential complications with nursing interventions.	**Classroom:** • Unit exam: One application and one analysis-level question included on test blueprint. **Clinical:** • Clinical evaluation tool to include competency. • Concept map with grading rubric.

Without a plan, the curriculum readily becomes "additive" and oversaturated with content.

The teaching-learning strategies provide information about how to teach the content at the appropriate level of thinking. On the lesson plan, faculty indicate the strategies used to teach content and thinking as well as any technology used to implement the curriculum through unit lessons.

Finally, the evaluation methods column of the lesson plan demonstrates how student achievement of the unit objectives will be measured. The test blueprint for development of test items links each item back to a unit objective and indicates the cognitive level of the test item. This demonstrates validity of the test; that is, the test is testing the content being taught as well as the level of thinking expected in that course as expressed through the unit objectives and course SLOs and competencies. These documents demonstrate internal consistency of the curriculum; that is, all parts of the curriculum relate.

Revise the Curriculum Based on Evaluation of Program Outcomes, Learner Needs, Societal and Health Care Trends, and Stakeholder Feedback

The information presented in this chapter reflects educational design principles; that is, all pieces of the curriculum are meaningful, serve a purpose, and fit together in a logical, consistent manner. All parts of the curriculum serve a purpose and are supportive of the other parts. Educational design principles, also known as instructional design, provide the basis for the total curriculum package. Faculty use educational principles, theory, and research when constructing the total curriculum package, which includes all curricular components. Educational research provides the best practices faculty can use as they implement the curriculum (Cannon & Boswell, 2012; Felver et al., 2010; Ironside & McNelis, 2010). A review of the educational literature provides an abundance of resources.

Two important factors faculty must consider when designing curriculum are content taught and characteristics of students. The curriculum delivers content to address learner needs by leveling according to the type of program—entry-level practical nursing, entry-level registered nursing, advanced practice nursing, and other graduate level coursework. Breaking down content and thinking into their component parts and determining the best approach to teaching is one aspect. For example, if the approach to teaching the content and thinking is conceptual, then theories that support conceptual learning such as constructivist or cognitive learning theory will be used.

The other aspect to consider when selecting which educational theories and research to use to deliver the curriculum is a knowledge of your students' characteristics. There are an array of characteristics to consider. Examples include age of the students, culture, fluency in the use of the English language, prior life experiences, prior educational experiences, and current life responsibilities. These characteristics may provide data to determine if a theory such as adult learning theory can be used to deliver the curriculum. Understanding the rationale for selecting educational principles, theories, and research to use in the design and implementation of the curriculum provides the evidence on which your approach is based (Erickson, 2008; Fink, 2013; Knowles, Holton, & Swanson, 2011; Schunk, 2012; Wiggins & McTighe, 2006).

Educational theory and instructional design principles continue to evolve. The main focus of face-to-face delivery of the curriculum is extended to include distance technologies. The design for the delivery of the curriculum via distance education (web-based, video, etc.) requires different considerations when the faculty and student are separated by time and distance. Faculty designing courses for delivery via distance education apply best practices that may be different from those previously used for classroom delivery (Ard & Valiga, 2009; Frith & Clark, 2012; Nelson, 2010).

An additional evolution in the design of the delivery of the curriculum relates to simulation. Designing simulation experiences requires additional strategies that may be new to faculty. It is important to use the literature when developing evidence-based strategies for delivering instruction via simulation (Jeffries, 2010; Jeffries, Settles, Milgrom, & Woolf, 2010).

The theoretical basis for the nursing curriculum requires ongoing faculty development. Most faculty are experts in a particular area of nursing practice and engage in ongoing continuing education related to that practice. This is critical to ensure societal and health care trends are part of the nursing curriculum. However, education is an equally important area of expertise for faculty. Ongoing development related to all aspects of curriculum development including educational theory, practice, instructional and learning activities, and evaluation methodologies is part of a continuing education process for nursing education faculty and administrators.

Revising the curriculum based on valuation of program outcomes is part of the program's assessment plan. This plan is addressed in the next section.

DESIGN, IMPLEMENT, AND EVALUATE THE PROGRAM ASSESSMENT PLAN

Another ongoing task for faculty is evaluating the effectiveness of the curriculum. Are the students achieving course SLOs and competencies as they move toward achieving program SLOs and competencies? Are the aggregate program outcome evaluation data at the level of expectations? The evaluation phase of curriculum is often an area that receives the least amount of attention, although it is equally important as the development and implementation phases.

Program Assessment Plan

A systematic process is used to determine if the program is functioning as intended. There are a number of aspects included in the assessment plan: (a) student achievement of course SLOs in the classroom, laboratory, and clinical; (b) achievement of expected levels on examinations such as the NCLEX and certification exams; (c) retention rate; (d) graduate and employer satisfaction with the educational preparation of the graduate for practice; and (e) employment rates. Figure 4.1 provides an overview of the process for a prelicensure nursing program.

Student Achievement of Course SLOs in the Classroom and the Clinical Settings

Student achievement of course SLOs in the classroom is often seen as difficult to measure. However, an aid for measuring SLOs is to ensure all information on the lesson plan is linked. The evaluation column provides the method of measuring student achievement of each unit lesson objective aligned to each course SLO and competency. The data collected from the evaluation methods are used to determine student achievement for each SLO. Box 4.1 provides an example process for measuring student learning related to course SLOs.

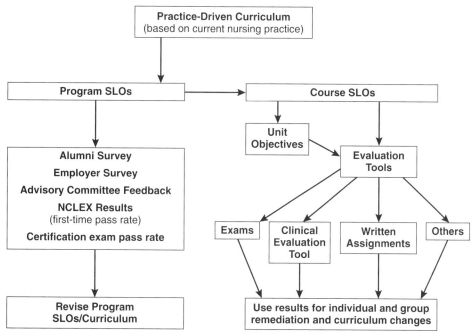

FIGURE 4.1 Curriculum Evaluation. Copyright © 2013, Linda Caputi, Inc. Used with permission.

BOX 4.1 Process for Evaluating Student Achievement of Course SLOs

Set an Expected Standard for Each Course SLO

Expected Level of Achievement
Students will score at 70 percent or higher on all test items related to course SLO 1.

Process
- The test blueprint provides a link to the unit objective that is linked to the course SLO.
- All items on an exam that are linked to course SLO 1 are aggregated to determine level of performance.
- If the combined percentage of all items for course SLO 1 is less than 70 percent, the expected level of achievement has not been met on that exam. The class needs additional instruction.
- The results of testing for items for course SLO 1 on *all* exams for the course are combined to determine if, at the end of the course, students have achieved at the 70 percent or higher level.
- If yes, the expected level of achievement has been met.
- If not, the expected level of achievement has not been met. Faculty must determine what changes in the curriculum and/or teaching-learning strategies should be made to correct the situation. Faculty should also offer additional instruction related to SLO 1 so current students will have the necessary information and thinking skills to progress to the next course.

This same process is used for each of the course SLOs. This example is related to classroom exams, but the process is used for evaluation methods for other assignments as well. For example, a scholarly paper assignment should directly align to specific course SLOs. The paper is then graded using a rubric for the various aspects of the assignment. The grading rubric provides information about student performance linked to the course SLOs addressed by the assignment. The data are then aggregated for all students completing the assignment to determine if the cohort has met the expected level of achievement set by faculty.

This process is also used for evaluation of clinical achievement of course SLOs. Faculty are accustomed to using clinical evaluation tools for individual student performance appraisal. However, that same data are not typically aggregated to determine whether the clinical experiences of each clinical group and of the cohort as a whole are meeting the expected levels of achievement. Aggregated data about the cohort as a whole are important to determine if the curriculum is functioning as intended.

Achievement of Expected Levels on Examinations such as the NCLEX and Certification Exams

The measures of graduate achievement of the program outcomes of NCLEX and certification exam pass rates are fairly objective. Although they are often used as a measure of program quality and achievement of program SLOs, recent practices using standardized exams as a gate for graduation from a prelicensure nursing program have confounded the NCLEX pass rates as a measure of a quality nursing program. According to Spurlock (2013, p. 7), "While artificially driving up licensure pass rates may protect a program from regulatory or accreditation actions, progression policies based on high-stakes testing do nothing to improve educational program quality and divert attention from the issues that could be impacting NCLEX-RN pass rates, including poor instructional quality, disruptive or inadequate learning environments, and lack of effective learning resources." If schools use a commercial standardized examination as a means to graduate only those students who the testing deems ready to pass the NCLEX, then the NCLEX results are not an accurate evaluation of program quality.

Retention Rate

The percentage of students who graduate from a nursing program is an important indicator of program quality. Generally speaking, students who are accepted into a nursing program are likely to have completed the program within 150 percent of the length of the program from entry into the first nursing course. Faculty again set an expected level of achievement. The established level should reflect student characteristics, history of student retention, and expectations of the parent organization. Retention rates have become increasingly important as the status of financial aid is affected when students do not advance or complete a program of study. Therefore, the curriculum must be constructed to be reasonable; that is, the program plan of study is designed to ensure the credit hours and weekly clock hours required are doable for students enrolled in the program. Additionally, faculty must consider the number of hours required for outside class study. Credit hours are calculated as one credit for three clock hours of work. Typically the credit hour calculation of one clock hour in a classroom theory session includes two additional clock hours of out-of-class study. Many clinical sessions are calculated at three clock hours of attendance for each one credit hour. This means the three clock hours for one credit hour are included as part of the clinical day. Therefore, there should be no out-of-clinical work expectations of the students; in so doing,

students are putting in more hours than needed to earn the credit. It is critical that faculty consider all these hours when determining the number of credit hours for each course and for the program total. Overloading students with more out-of-class work than is reasonable for the credit hours earned can result in student failure and a high attrition rate.

Graduate and Employer Satisfaction and Employment Rates

Collecting data to determine graduate and employer satisfaction with the nursing program and employment rates is often achieved through the use of a survey. Graduates and employers complete surveys with questions directly related to program SLOs. Both graduates and employers should evaluate the extent to which the new graduate is able to use the knowledge and thinking skills acquired through achievement of the program SLOs in their first nursing position. The value of the program SLOs should also be evaluated. Do the program SLOs represent what is currently important to nursing practice? Are they meeting the needs of the graduate? Do they represent societal needs and current healthcare trends? Only the graduates and their employers know the answers to these questions. Therefore, it is important to implement strategies resulting in a high return rate for these surveys. This often presents one of the greatest barriers to measurement of these program outcomes. Nursing programs have instituted many tactics in an attempt to experience a high return rate. Mailing surveys is perhaps the least effective strategy. Direct calls to graduates, personal visits to employers, and, more recently, the use of social media have increased return rates, although requiring additional time and labor, both of which are difficult to attain especially if the school is experiencing financial tightening. However, measuring program outcomes is not a place to decrease efforts to cut costs. If program outcomes are not measured, there is no evidence the program is effective and no data to guide ongoing program improvement.

Analyze Results of Program Evaluation

Data that reflect the level of achievement of program SLOs and program outcomes are used to improve the nursing program. The full range of possibilities exists depending on the results. Because curriculum has many facets, the data must be analyzed to determine what specifically to address to improve program effectiveness. Elements of the curriculum that may be changed based on the data include (a) student admission requirements, (b) grading scale, (c) sequencing of nursing courses, (d) required nonnursing courses, (e) teaching strategies, (f) evaluation methods, (g) content taught, and (h) integration of clinical reasoning at all levels. This is not an all-inclusive list. It is obvious that data from evaluation methods are used to improve all aspects of a nursing program. Analyses of the data by faculty and nursing administration provide the basis for these improvement discussions. Any and all changes made must be evaluated to determine their effectiveness. Therefore, program evaluation is ongoing.

IMPLEMENT CURRICULAR REVISIONS USING APPROPRIATE CHANGE THEORIES AND STRATEGIES

The implication of the discussion of this chapter is that faculty are best positioned to be the leader of curriculum development, implementation, evaluation, and revision. Faculty are at the forefront of the educational process and the nursing profession and are, therefore, the best prepared to engage in curriculum work. Curriculum is the responsibility of all faculty, and all faculty should be informed and aware of the total curriculum and all related processes. Often faculty work in silos, meaning each faculty member teaches his or her own course and is unable to discuss how other courses fit into the curriculum. It is important that faculty take ownership of the entire curriculum, be knowledgeable about the entire curriculum, and understand how each course contributes to the overall success of the curriculum. As faculty design the courses they teach, that design process must support the program SLOs and the overall mission and purpose of the nursing program. The faculty work as a team and each individual team member contributes equally to the curriculum.

COLLABORATE WITH COMMUNITY AND CLINICAL PARTNERS TO SUPPORT EDUCATIONAL GOALS

The curriculum is reflective of the external nursing and health care environment. As faculty work together to ensure a current, rigorous nursing program, they also work with community and clinical partners to ensure educational outcomes are appropriate for current practice. Developing partnerships with health care agencies to ensure not just clinical placement but also an alignment of thinking related to clinical experiences is important. Additionally, in the current health care environment, nursing programs can no longer work independently. Ironside and McNelis (2010) advise that new clinical models must foster partnerships among faculty, students, schools, clinical agencies, staff nurses, and preceptors with the intent to align clinical learning with contemporary practice and health care needs. Nursing schools must work together, "sharing resources to prepare the next generation of nurses" (IOM, 2011, p. 174).

Practice Test Questions

1. The nursing faculty are developing competency statements for students who will participate in a clinical practicum immediately prior to graduation. Which statement is most reflective of this plan?

A. Develop basic plans of care using the nursing process for patients with common alterations in health status.

B. Prioritize care for assigned patients and delegate as appropriate to assistive personnel.

C. Organize and manage care for assigned patients assisting other students as needed.

D. Organize and deliver care according to established priorities for patients experiencing common medical-surgical problems.

2. Faculty decide to revise a 25-year-old curriculum and are developing a list of tasks. Which task should be completed first?

A. Investigate the knowledge, skills, and attitudes needed for current nursing practice.

B. Update the theoretical framework of the old curriculum on which to build the new curriculum.

C. Decide if a concept-based curriculum is best for the program.

D. Poll the clinical agencies about their expectations of graduates.

3. A new nursing faculty is assigned to develop an adult health course as part of the curriculum revision process. Which statement best guides the faculty's development of the course?

A. Compare the course with a similar course in a colleague's school to determine if content is the same.

B. Follow the textbook when developing course outlines to ensure all content in the book is covered.

C. Understand faculty are the experts so the content included should be determined solely by the faculty teaching the course.

D. Ensure the content addresses course student learning outcomes that build on those of the prerequisite nursing courses.

4. Which statement best represents the overall purpose of a program assessment plan?

A. Determine if the faculty teaching strategies are effective.

B. Determine if the program is functioning as intended.

C. Provide information about student characteristics as the basis for determining admission criteria.

D. Provide data on which to develop a student retention program.

5. The director of the nursing program is chairing the meeting with the advisory council consisting of clinical partners and others interested in the nursing program. Which question would be best for the director to ask of the committee members to receive input for curriculum revision?

A. What changes in health care do you see as important for the nurses in your facility?

B. What would you like us to teach in the program?

C. Are you satisfied with our graduates?

D. Do the nurses on your units find the students helpful during their clinical rotations?

References

Accreditation Commission for Education in Nursing, Inc. (ACEN). (2013). *The NLNAC accreditation manual.* Atlanta, GA: Author.

American Nurses Association (ANA). (2008). *Position statement on professional role competence.* Washington, DC: American Nurses Publishing.

Anderson, L. W., Krathwohl, D. R., Airasian, P. W., Cruikshank, K. A., Mayer, R. E., Pintrich, P. R., Rathis, J., & Wittrock, M. C. (2001). *A taxonomy for learning, teaching, and assessing: A revision of Bloom's taxonomy of educational objectives.* New York: Longman.

Ard, N., & Valiga, T. (2009). *Clinical nursing education: Current reflections.* New York: National League for Nursing.

Cannon, S., & Boswell, C. (2012). *Evidence-based teaching in nursing: A foundation for educators.* Sudbury, MA: Jones & Bartlett.

Caputi, L. (Ed.). (2010). *Curriculum design and development.* In L. Caputi (Ed.), *Teaching nursing: The art and science* (2nd ed., Vol. 1, pp. 367–402). Glen Ellyn, IL: DuPage Press.

Commission on Collegiate Nursing Education (CCNE). (2013). *Standards for accreditation of baccalaureate and graduate nursing programs.* Washington, DC: Author. Retrieved from www.aacn.nche.edu/ccne-accreditation/ Standards-Amended-2013.pdf

Erickson, H. L. (2008). *Stirring the head, heart, and soul: Redefining curriculum, instruction, and concept-based learning* (3rd ed.). Thousand Oaks, CA: Corwin.

Felver, L., Gaines, B., Heims, M., Lasater, K., Laustsen, G., Lynch, M.,...Tanner, C. (2010). *Best practices in teaching and learning in nursing education.* New York: National League for Nursing.

Fink, L. D. (2013). *Creating significant learning experiences: An integrated approach to designing college courses, revised and updated.* San Francisco: Jossey-Bass.

Frith, K., & Clark, D. (2012). *Distance education in nursing* (3rd ed.). New York: Springer.

Giddens, J. F., & Brady, D. P. (2007). Rescuing nursing education from content saturation: The case for a concept-based curriculum. *Nursing Education Perspectives, 46*(2), 65–69.

Halstead, J. (2007). *Nurse educator competencies: Creating an evidence-based practice for nurse educators.* New York: National League for Nursing.

Institute of Medicine (IOM). (2011). *The future of nursing: Leading change, advancing health.* Washington, DC: National Academies Press.

Ironside, P. M. (2004). "Covering content" and teaching thinking: Deconstructing the additive curriculum. *Journal of Nursing Education, 43*(1), 5–12.

Ironside, P. M., & McNelis, A. M. (2010). *Clinical education in prelicensure nursing programs: Results from an NLN national survey.* New York: National League for Nursing.

Jeffries, P. R. (2010). *Simulation in nursing education: From conceptualization to evaluation.* New York: National League for Nursing.

Jeffries, P. R., Settles, J., Milgrom, L., & Woolf, S. K. (2010). Using simulations: Guidelines and challenges. In L. Caputi (Ed.), *Teaching nursing: The art and science* (2nd ed., Vol. 2, pp. 56–80). Glen Ellyn, IL: DuPage Press.

Knowles, M. S., Holton, E. F., & Swanson, R. A. (2011). *The adult learner.* Burlington, MA: Elsevier.

National League for Nursing (NLN). (2010). *Outcomes and competencies for graduates of practical/vocational, diploma, associate degree, baccalaureate, master's, practice doctorate, and research doctorate programs in nursing.* New York: Author.

Nelson, R. (2010). Distance education technology: Implications for nursing education. In L. Caputi (Ed.), *Teaching nursing: The art and science* (2nd ed., Vol. 2, pp. 599–740). Glen Ellyn, IL: DuPage Press.

Schunk, D. H. (2012). *Learning theories: An educational perspective* (6th ed.). Upper Saddle River, NJ: Pearson.

Spurlock, D. (2013). The promise and peril of high-stake tests in nursing education. *Journal of Nursing Regulation, 4*(1), 4–8.

Wiggins, G., & McTighe, J. (2006). *Understanding by design.* Upper Saddle River, NJ: Pearson.

5

Pursue Systematic Self-Evaluation and Improvement in the Academic Nurse Educator Role

Wanda Blaser Bonnel, PhD, RN, GNP-BC, ANEF

The CNE Test Plan Lists the Following for the Area of Pursue Systematic Self-Evaluation and Improvement in the Academic Nurse Educator Role:

5. Pursue Systematic Self-Evaluation and Improvement in the Academic Nurse Educator Role

A. Engage in activities that promote one's socialization to the role

B. Maintain membership in professional organizations

C. Participate actively in professional organizations through committee work and/or leadership roles

D. Demonstrate a commitment to lifelong learning

E. Participate in professional development opportunities that increase one's effectiveness in the role

F. Manage the teaching, scholarship, and service demands as influenced by the requirements of the institutional setting

G. Use feedback gained from self, peer, learner, and administrative evaluation to improve role effectiveness

H. Practice according to legal and ethical standards relevant to higher education and nursing education

I. Mentor and support faculty colleagues in the role of an academic nurse educator

J. Engage in self-reflection to improve teaching practices

Nurse educators recognize that their role is multidimensional and that an ongoing commitment to develop and maintain competence in the role is essential (NLN, 2012a, p. 20).

The nursing faculty role is multidimensional. The role requires faculty to develop and maintain competence in venues such as clinician, educator, and scholar. This competency includes components that are interactive and supportive. Ongoing quality improvement in the faculty role is a central theme uniting these.

Quality improvement has gained recent emphasis within the culture of safety and quality in health care (IOM, 2003, 2011). Quality improvement serves as a basic problem-solving model that involves systematically assessing situations and implementing plans to address identified problems or gaps. It involves addressing the big picture with systems thinking in mind. Although the literature is replete with articles describing clinical quality improvement projects, the quality improvement concept is important in education as well. Quality work in academia is described as activities that are organized and dedicated to improve the quality of education and research (Massey, Graham, & Short, 2007). Quality improvement models are relevant for addressing courses and programs as well as useful for career enhancement. Accountability and ongoing improvement are key components of quality improvement (Kurtzman & Johnson, 2012).

Research and best evidence are also key components of quality improvement. Best evidence, in addition to available research support, includes best summary evidence from respected organizations. Of note, if research literature and best evidence are limited, well-developed theories serve as guides to help organize educator activities. Particularly relevant are "big picture" models useful in mapping out teaching and career plans and with systems models such as Donabedian's (1982) model of structure, process, and outcomes. Theories such as Knowles, Holton, and Swanson's (1998) "Adult Learner" and Finks' (2003) integrated learning model are theory examples useful in guiding teaching-learning practices. Boyer's (1990) scholarship model and Myers and Jaeger's (2012) quality improvement model also have relevance in career planning.

ENGAGE IN ACTIVITIES THAT PROMOTE ONE'S SOCIALIZATION TO THE ROLE

The academic setting presents a unique culture. Learning the role expectations and strategies to become socialized to this setting is instrumental in becoming a successful part of the culture. Socialization extends beyond the nursing program to include the college and the larger professional community. Across settings, roles can include citizens of the college and of the profession. Within these roles the focus will at times be on varied roles or activities, such as administrator, course leader, coach or mentor, peer colleague, or team member.

Theories, Evidence, and Tools

Socialization is considered an ongoing process where individuals learn values, norms, skills, and behaviors appropriate to a social position. For role socialization, individuals take on the habits and skills needed to successfully participate in the environmental context (Blake, Ashforth, Sluss, & Saks, 2007). In part socialization is based on role theory, roles based on social or professional norms, the organizational context, personal characteristics, skills, and role interpretation (Biddle, 1979). Common related terms include role conflict or incompatibility (faculty lacking time, skill, or needed education); role ambiguity (lacking clarity on the role); role stress (vague obligations that are difficult, conflicting, or impossible to meet); or role strain (roles that create frustration, tension, or anxiety). Role socialization includes spending time getting to know the culture. It is also guided by change theory as new ways and systems are sought to be engaged in the profession. Strategies to support role transitions and socialization include learning the setting, getting oriented to the system, and building on the familiar.

Learning Your Setting

As noted, part of socialization includes a good academic match initially and clarity on the type of role in which faculty are employed. Once a setting has been chosen, questions to help learn the setting include the National League for Nursing's (NLN, 2006) guide to the healthy work environment. This document provides a series of questions that can be adapted to assess a new environment. Developed from a national survey of faculty satisfaction and productivity and an extensive literature review, the report provides sample questions in sections that include "Role Preparation and Professional Development"; "Collegial Environment"; and "Workload and Scholarship." An example would be questions specific to role preparation and development that relate to asking about an academic setting's resources for development and how faculty gain assistance in career planning.

Get Oriented to the Setting

Culture shock in academia can occur if a good orientation and mentoring program does not exist (Kahanov, Eberman, Yoder, & Kahanov, 2012). Ask questions to determine if a faculty orientation process is in place and what that means. To better learn about an academic system, seek assistance in creating a map of faculty and staff colleagues and their roles. In this map, include expected relationships or a responsibility chart that outlines team member roles and how each role relates within the larger team. Learn informal and formal communication channels, identifying those with strong power and influence, and seek opportunities to learn from them (Bolman & Deal, 2008).

Good communication and good use of resource persons are starting points in learning about a work setting. Advocate for a mentor, and seek tours and orientation opportunities. Identify resource persons and seek opportunities to work with them. It is important to clarify early on when there is uncertainty as to what to do in a particular situation, such as when using record keeping in electronic learning systems and the phone numbers for technologies support.

Build on Familiar Connections

Many new educators are transitioning from clinical roles to faculty roles. Recalling past teaching experiences such as patient education and roles in mentoring new clinical staff can help inform new academic educator roles. The adult education principles used in these situations are helpful to transition into teaching in a new academic setting. As each new academic system brings new expectations, new support systems such as faculty mentors and trusted colleagues will be needed.

These same concepts that are useful in the academic nursing program extend to socialization to larger college venues and professional organizations. Seek active roles in each venue where you can observe, participate, and learn.

MAINTAIN MEMBERSHIP IN PROFESSIONAL ORGANIZATIONS; PARTICIPATE ACTIVELY IN PROFESSIONAL ORGANIZATIONS THROUGH COMMITTEE WORK AND/OR LEADERSHIP ROLES

Membership in professional organizations has always been an important aspect of lifelong learning for nurses. Membership in professional nursing education organizations is equally important for the nurse educator. The multifaceted role of the nurse educator requires expertise in a practice area as well as in nursing education. Therefore, membership in professional organizations is twofold: membership in clinical practice organizations and membership in nursing education organizations such as the National League for Nursing. Nursing education has experienced rapid changes over the past decade. Obvious changes are the expanded use of simulation and the Internet to deliver courses. Less obvious, but equally important, are other changes such as approaches to curriculum development, overarching concepts that provide the basis for competency-based nursing education, and the use of research to form an evidence base for nursing education. These are just a few areas that have experienced change over the past decade and many others emerge yearly through the published reports of the Institute of Medicine, the National League for Nursing, and other influential organizations. Membership in professional organizations as a conduit for delivery of these and many other changes provides a method for continuous quality improvement for nursing faculty.

Service to professional organizations is another important aspect of membership. Professional nursing organizations provide opportunities to promote career advancement via varied leadership roles. These can result in professional satisfaction as you participate and give back to the organization and its causes. There is particular value in networking and information exchange via these specialty organizations. They provide opportunities for following and addressing trends and concerns of the specialty. The value in organizational membership involves participating in meaningful activities and gaining practice with leadership activities that can also be applied to the work setting. As an active member of these associations, you are also helping to accomplish the work of the profession (Shinn, 2013).

DEMONSTRATE A COMMITMENT TO LIFELONG LEARNING

Lifelong learning involves a commitment to remain current within the rapidly changing health care world as well as changing needs or roles in nursing education. A commitment to lifelong learning requires efficiency because as nurse educators this typically means commitment to updating on a regular basis including both clinical topic areas in which you are teaching and best teaching-learning practices.

Theories, Evidence, and Tools

Lifelong learning is consistent with the theory of constructivism (Glaserfeld, 1989) and constructing learning to fit with the needs and roles in nursing. Benner's (1984) novice to expert strategies can be used as a guide to map quality improvement plans. Useful tools to guide lifelong learning include reflective self-assessment, self-directed learning, and mapping out learning needs.

Reflective Self-Assessment

Reflective self-assessment involves knowing yourself, including determination of what you know related to your career role and what you still need to know (McBride, 2010). Reflection provides an opportunity to engage one's thinking specific to experiences and to learn from these experiences, reflecting on a problem or a positive incident to consider what has been learned (Schon, 1987). Self-assessment involves assessing or evaluating against some type of standard or rubric. For example, as you review this book, the National League for Nursing (NLN) competencies serve as a summary of educational best practices and a type of standard. You can assess your strengths and needed areas of work related to each of the competencies.

Self-Directed Learning

Self-directed learning skills are important tools, not only for faculty but also for the students being taught. Self-directed learning has a range of meanings. For example, in an educator course the instructor may provide an active learning assignment or a menu of activities and let each person choose those that are most relevant and meaningful. The idea is to allow opportunities to learn about concepts in ways that best fit each person's own life or career patterns. Tools and resources for the self-directed learner such as contracting and journaling have been summarized by Hiemstra (2010). In a rapidly changing health care and nursing education world, these are necessary skills to maintain currency and organize vast amounts of information.

Mapping

Mapping out a career plan is a useful starting point for lifelong, self-directed learning. It begins with self-assessment and involves creating a career plan or road map flowing from personal objectives. In other words, for each career objective the nurse educator might ask:

- What related education will I need to gain?
- How will I apply this learning?
- How will I evaluate success?

Writing out a plan can include a reflective component. This reflection serves to:

1. Keep you focused
2. Reinforce action steps
3. Assist you as you build on your planned pathway.

McBride (2010) describes this mapping as orchestrating a career. It evolves to a focus on outcomes that can be named and described on a curriculum vitae (CV), rather than a listing of activities.

PARTICIPATE IN PROFESSIONAL DEVELOPMENT OPPORTUNITIES THAT INCREASE ONE'S EFFECTIVENESS IN THE ROLE

Professional development involves strategically planning a career and considering what role development activities are needed. It is an active process that plays a role in faculty motivation and promoting ongoing quality improvement for faculty at all levels. It also can connect faculty across and within disciplines to promote increased satisfaction with the academic experience (Altany, 2012). Professional development opportunities along with faculty mentors are key components of the academic career journey (Penn, Wilson, & Rosseter, 2008).

Efficient and effective strategies for development support not just a clinical specialty but also scholarship and teaching roles. Staying current with trends in a clinical specialty and the best evidence about the subject matter of assigned courses that are being taught means staying current with the best evidence for teaching and learning.

Theories, Evidence, and Tools

Theories of adult education and strategic planning can be of value when planning further education for specific roles. The theory of adult education presented in Knowles et al. (1998) can provide direction in packaging programs that are relevant and engaging for personal development. Tools and approaches in role development include strategic planning and use of both formal and informal educational approaches.

Strategic Planning: Your Education/Development

Strategic planning involves charting a course relevant to the roles being pursued. As you identify what you want to do with your career, you begin to identify the types of education you will need to make that happen. Faculty effectiveness involves knowing what education and role development activities are needed for a career. It involves reflecting on the personal philosophy that directs a person's goals and plans, and then laying out activities to gain these. Because time is a limited quantity, it is good to choose efficient approaches to professional development.

Formal Approaches to Development

Often professional development involves advancing education. This involves making choices about what type of education program will best meet specific needs. Common approaches include the educator or nursing practice doctorate and the research-focused philosophy degree in nursing or a related field. Fellowships provide a way to document further expertise (McBride, 2010). Educational choices of best programs are those that relate to your own interests and the needs of your chosen academic setting.

For those who hold a terminal degree, certification provides a way to document further expertise and clinical advancement. For example, clinical competencies can be documented via certifications such as those developed by the American Nurses Association or other specialty organizations. Educator competencies can be documented via certification with the Certified Nurse Educator examination consistent with the NLN competencies (NLN, 2012a). Consistent with lifelong learning, as situations or career plans change, ongoing education is key.

Informal Approaches to Role Development/Continuing Education

As lifelong learners, attaining good resources to keep up with the rapidly changing world of health care practice and education is key. This involves reading the journals and participating in formal or informal journal clubs or related activities. An efficient personal system might involve staying current with several respected journals. Numerous nursing education journals exist such as the NLN's *Nursing Education Perspectives,* which is a leader in nursing education research. Current issues in higher education are reported in journals such as the *Chronicle of Higher Education.* Clinical newsletters and online resources such as Tomorrow's Professor or drEd are valuable resources to scan for relevant educator topics. Additionally, peruse other clinical journals for relevant contributions to specific specialties.

Other educational venues for lifelong learning in nursing education are provided by specialty organizations and clinical or academic work settings. Specialty organizations often provide resources for the educator. For example, the NLN (2008a) provides broad initiatives, such as informatics competencies, with tools for helping students learn to use patient data via electronic health records for quality improvement. The NLN is also a leader in providing evidence-based simulation education and care of the elderly. Other broad areas that help with professional development include seeking educational opportunities across the clinical setting or academic campus and learning from other professionals as they build the educational component of their CV.

Completing projects, presentations, and publications also serves as a form of education. McBride (2010) summarized that scholarly publications beyond research are key. For example, sharing evaluative projects that you develop provides opportunities for others to learn and for you to gain respect in that arena.

MANAGE THE TEACHING, SCHOLARSHIP, AND SERVICE DEMANDS AS INFLUENCED BY THE REQUIREMENTS OF THE INSTITUTIONAL SETTING

Expectations can be high for those in the role of educator. Some find that fulfilling multiple role expectations, typically including education, service, and research, can be very challenging and at times even unrealistic. As noted, academic life or priorities will be different in an institution with a research focus versus one with a teaching focus. Approaches for balancing include being strategic and learning the realities of unique academic organizations.

Theories, Evidence, and Tools

In addition to quality improvement and strategic planning models, Boyer's (1990) model is important when considering direction on balancing scholarly products. Boyer describes the importance of acknowledging faculty educational scholarship as well as clinical research. His classic framework for documenting educational scholarship includes teaching, application, integration, and discovery. Boyer's framework provides a model for helping faculty not only share educational products with others, but also to reflect on and continue to improve teaching products. Benner's (1984) model of novice to expert can also be relevant in showing advancing expertise via product development.

Service is a common academic role along with scholarship and teaching. Although scholarship and teaching are discussed in other chapters of this book, examples of service roles are addressed here.

Balancing Academic Service

Service is identified in multiple ways in academia. Typically this first involves service to the academic organization and then service to the larger community, both professional communities and patient populations. Service definitions vary by types of settings. For example, in some cases service may be defined to include volunteer activities only and others may include paid service such as clinical practice. Service to the broader community is often considered a form of giving back to the community. To gain the most value, Cardinal (2013) recommends selecting service roles that mesh with authentic service work that relates to your specialty interests.

Committee work, such as evaluation, curriculum, promotion or tenure, and student admissions or progression committees, is often considered service to a program or school. These also provide new faculty with information about how the nursing program and institutions work.

Balancing via Role Consolidation

Role consolidation that maximizes faculty interests and minimizes workload is considered an important practice (Bartels, 2007). Role consolidation refers to combining roles. For example, if opportunities to choose committee memberships exist, it is often helpful to identify a committee related to specific interests. If focusing on specific teaching interests, it may be useful to be part of a curriculum or evaluation committee. These committee work opportunities may provide ideas for your own course planning and best evaluation practices. By obtaining a role to help monitor or improve the quality of the academic program, you can gain insights for your own teaching.

Balancing with Your Team

You and your colleague team can also create opportunities by "dividing and conquering." Whether your team is nursing or interprofessional, there is value in working together on project completion and considering multiple authors for project dissemination. In making the most of your team, the following questions can be helpful:

1. Who are the key people on your team?
2. What strategies are you using to collaborate with clinical and teaching colleagues?
3. What do you do to promote a smooth working relationship and engagement with your team?
4. What do you do if team members are less than supportive?

Balancing Self-Development

Balancing also involves recognizing that a career is meant to last a lifetime and that all activities and projects do not need to be planned and completed all at once (McBride, 2010). Balancing often means assessing and planning one's activities from a big picture focus; for example, focusing on select components of the common educator roles (teaching, service, research, and scholarship) during different semesters, years, or even different career points. For example, several years can focus on scholarship and research, and other years might focus on expert educator roles and curriculum development types of projects. Timelines can involve a day, a month, or 5- and 10-year plans. Consider applying the following questions to all your activities, even your daily activities:

1. What is most needed?
2. Where should the most time be spent?
3. Do schedule alterations need to be made?

Balancing Self-Care

Balancing also involves taking care of oneself. Dealing with role stress and strain in the academic setting requires coping strategies, such as self-advocacy, to meet mutually agreed goals and advocate for a win-win situation. Other health promotion strategies are critical as well, as you care for yourself, you model healthy behaviors for patients and students. Balancing roles involves creating a timeline including what you need and want to do in a manageable format. The manageable format can vary by career or family responsibilities. Balance in your career can be summarized in your professional portfolio, with each chapter contributing to the whole as developed over time.

USE FEEDBACK GAINED FROM SELF, PEER, LEARNER, AND ADMINISTRATIVE EVALUATION TO IMPROVE ROLE EFFECTIVENESS

Just as feedback is used to evaluate educational programs to support quality improvement, it is also used to evaluate and provide guidance for faculty. Processing feedback involves being open, listening, receiving, and using the evaluation data to enhance clinical and academic activities and roles.

Theories, Evidence, and Tools

Communication models are a major part of feedback, with listening as an active process. Feedback is considered communication of information that assists an individual to reflect and interact with the information to construct self-knowledge and set further goals. Feedback needs to be acknowledged and used appropriately to be effective (Bonnel, 2008; Bonnel & Boehm, 2011). Feedback is not considered a final grade of work, but rather a formative assessment for improving teaching and academic efforts. It gauges accomplishments and allows an individual to take further responsibility for ongoing improvement.

Feedback is used to increase effectiveness in diverse educator roles across an individual's career. At certain points, some types of feedback may be more important than others, depending on the role's focus. For example, feedback related to teaching and classroom presentation skills is different from feedback on scholarly work such as a grant proposal.

Triangulation of Methods

The concept of triangulation is an important concept when considering the value of feedback. Triangulation involves gaining feedback from multiple evaluators (self, peers, learners, administration) through use of multiple methods and approaches. Triangulation increases the credibility and validity of feedback results.

Using Student Ratings of Teaching as Feedback

A common method for acquiring feedback in academia is from students via class and course evaluations. Students provide their perspective on the value of select class features. McKeachie and Svinicki (2013) note the value of gaining student feedback on classes early in the semester, rather than waiting only until the end, is to provide time to use the feedback and make teaching or course improvements. For example, when teaching a class, a best practice includes asking for fast feedback from students. Fast feedback forms ask students several questions related to class learning and satisfaction. There is particular value in the approach because it provides rapid confirmation of what is working or what needs to be fixed in a classroom session. If used for multiple teaching sessions, fast feedback helps identify larger patterns of classroom strengths and weaknesses. McKeachie and Svinicki also recommend review of fast feedback summaries with students including discussing with them what changes have been made based on their input. This process, coupled with an end of semester course evaluation, helps provide a summary of both faculty strengths and further development needs.

End of the semester feedback from students using a standardized format is a common approach to course evaluation. Although debate exists about the amount of weight to place on the final student course evaluations, Benton and Cashin (2009) provide an overview of research and issues related to student ratings of teaching. They summarize that in general, student ratings tend to be statistically reliable, valid, and relatively free from bias.

Feedback from students can be coupled with feedback from other sources and summarized in faculty yearly reviews. This process provides a quality improvement opportunity to summarize the faculty's responses to any problem areas. Also, if student evaluations are troubling, it is helpful to consult with a trusted experienced colleague or mentor to deal with the disappointing student evaluations. Strategies for further quality improvement can be shared by this individual (McKeachie & Svinicki, 2013).

Feedback from Peers and Administrators

Peers and administrators can provide additional useful perspectives on a teacher's teaching role. The concepts of peer assessment and peer review are used interchangeably throughout the literature. Peer review is described as an inter-active process of providing feedback to peers based on specific criteria with the intent to promote professional growth. It is a process of communicating evaluative information that has been collected and interpreted within a comfortable environ-ment created for this exchange (Boehm & Bonnel, 2010). Constructive peer feed-back is often facilitated via a systematic, organized process typically incorporating a standardized rubric. Schools often have peer feedback forms available, or these can be found in the literature. These provide additional data to incorporate into annual summary reviews.

Self-Assessment

Self-assessment is a useful feedback strategy. McKeachie and Svinicki (2013) note that a benefit to being an educator is always having something more to learn about oneself. He advocates self-reflection as a central tool in determining where one is professionally and what is needed. Bailey (1981), in an early work, advocated that faculty make a recording of their classroom teaching and use a rubric to self-assess classroom teaching strengths and weaknesses. This self-assessment goes beyond the teaching content to include nonverbal and verbal cues for engaging students in learning as well as myriad other teaching techniques the faculty may have used during the session.

PRACTICE ACCORDING TO LEGAL AND ETHICAL STANDARDS RELEVANT TO HIGHER EDUCATION AND NURSING EDUCATION

Unique and varied ethical and legal issues are common themes throughout health professions' educational settings. In addition to teaching students important ethical and legal principles that guide their clinical practice with patients, this competency focuses on the educator's use of these tools with students in academic settings.

Theories, Evidence, and Tools

Sound ethical and legal principles are used to develop and apply academic poli-cies. The familiar ethical principles of justice (being fair to all); autonomy (all individuals have rights); and beneficence (do no harm) are relevant principles in work with students. In addition to these common principles, a classic ref-erence from the American Association of Higher Education's (1996) "Ethical Principles for College and University Teaching" provides a summary of specific ethical issues to which the educator is mindful. These ethical principles provide guidance on issues dealing with sensitive topics in health professions educa-tion, cultural sensitivity issues, and incivility issues. Treating all individuals with respect is a key theme.

Legal issues include student rights and responsibilities as well as faculty guidelines for achieving and promoting these. Legal documents and resources applied when teaching nursing include the students' right to privacy, the Fam-ily Educational Rights and Privacy Act, students with disabilities (Americans with Disabilities Act), Health Insurance Portability and Accountability Act, stu-dent clinical safety issues, and legal aspects of documentation and record keep-ing. Students have the right to due process; this includes being familiar with students' rights to grievance and appeal processes. Although faculty have legal guidelines in existing policies and laws, Gaberson and Oermann (2010) note that legal counsel should be sought related to student-specific legal questions or problems.

Being Proactive

Being familiar with and sharing with students guiding documents prior to problem development is key to promoting professional student behaviors. Best approaches include proactive engagement of students. Important documents that provide guidance include student handbooks; course syllabi and policies; program academic integrity policies and honor codes; and academic and professional standards. Also important are policies in place by clinical agencies and the clinical agreements that outline student, faculty, and agency rights and responsibilities. Being proactive by helping students understand these policies can prevent later problems; they also provide direction for how faculty can best respond if there are challenges during implementation. Guidelines from national organizations such as the student focused National Student Nurses' Association (www.nsna.org/) also provide resources such as the "Bill of Rights and Responsibilities for Students of Nursing" and the "Code of Academic and Clinical Conduct: A Code for Nursing Students." The best times to be proactive include the beginning of programs and course orientations with regularly scheduled reminders to students.

Common Faculty Challenges

Common challenges in academia include being fair and consistent, promoting academic integrity, and promoting student professionalism in emerging areas, such as social networking. A proactive approach as noted is valuable.

BEING FAIR IN STUDENT EVALUATION

Some of the most common issues faculty deal with relate to fairness in evaluations of classroom and clinical work. Being fair and equitable in treatment of students includes having a fair grading policy for classroom, laboratory, and clinical settings. It is crucial to be honest, clear, and objective when grading in this high-stakes arena. Students should receive a clear explanation about grading of assignments while providing fair evaluations in all settings. As described by the NLN (2012b) fair testing document, evidence from multiple sources is needed for a fair evaluation. Although important across situations, this is particularly relevant when high-stakes testing is used.

Clinical settings present unique challenges and opportunities. The advent of high-technology learning labs provides valuable opportunities for a more standard clinical evaluation, such as skill check-offs with rubrics that promote student safety in actual clinical environments. It is important to establish interrater reliability for these evaluations when multiple raters evaluate students.

PROMOTING ACADEMIC INTEGRITY

Proactive strategies also promote academic integrity (Tippitt et al., 2009). Proactive strategies include:

1. Require students to sign pledges to engage in honesty
2. Create a safe environment that helps students feel secure enough to share actual or potential problems
3. Identify specific assignment approaches and strategies to help avoid plagiarism
4. Consider using tools such as a code of ethics documents in postconference discussions
5. Engage students in developing group resources such as specific civility documents.

If, after instituting proactive strategies, reactive strategies become necessary to deal with abuses of academic integrity, the following are useful:

1. Use ongoing, clear communication, including both written and verbal formats that document specific incidents as well as counseling efforts
2. Define the problem behaviors and appropriate responses (i.e., student smoking is very different from intentionally being rough with a patient)
3. Align the penalty to fit the offense
4. Use reasonable warnings with remediation opportunities
5. Contract for improved student outcomes (including written consequences)
6. Be prepared for discussions with students about problem behaviors with documentation included.

Again, recall that these reactive approaches involve using school resources as guides for enforcing expectations.

BEING FAIR IN DEALING WITH CHALLENGING STUDENT BEHAVIORS

As faculty focus on student competency and patient safety, it can be particularly frustrating to be confronted with issues such as tardiness or student rudeness. Remember to focus first on proactive strategies to prevent these behaviors, then use fair, reasonable, reactive strategies for dealing with problem behaviors. An example of ongoing interest is the increasing use of technology for social networking. The challenges for students to stay safe, legal, and ethical online are many. As students share enthusiasm, or try to be helpful, in their new nursing role, online settings provide many potential problems. Students must understand their behaviors on their seemingly private pages are actually public and require the same professional standards of patient privacy and confidentiality (NCSBN, 2011). Appropriate policies and discussions can help prevent student missteps.

Maintaining faculty professional behavior related to socialization with students is part of the AAHE's (1996) guidelines. Maintaining a professional student-faculty relationship involves thoughtful reflection on whether or how much socialization on a regular basis is appropriate. Faculty can strive to listen to their students without getting immersed and then model a comfortable professional relationship.

MENTOR AND SUPPORT FACULTY COLLEAGUES IN THE ROLE OF AN ACADEMIC NURSE EDUCATOR

Mentoring needs and approaches vary throughout an academic career. Mentoring extends throughout a career, not just at the beginning, and also can vary depending on the nature of the educational setting. At early career points, mentors help the new faculty to learn the ways of a program and of teaching. Concerns about "fitting in" the setting or academic milieu have been noted as a significant novice faculty stressor (Sawatzky & Enns, 2009). Although mentoring barriers can result from limited time and faculty support for mentoring, mentoring can be especially helpful in understanding the unique culture of academic institutions (Slimmer, 2012).

As faculty progress from novice to expert in select clinical and teaching areas, the time will arrive to help support and mentor others. Mentor and mentee roles may coexist as the mentee may have expertise to share with a more seasoned faculty member who then shares his or her expertise with the mentee. Taking on the mentoring role involves a self-assessment about strengths that faculty can offer as well as seeking a good match with a mentee.

Theories, Evidence, and Tools

A clear communication model that attends to message and sender or receiver variables is central to good mentoring. Both informal and formal mentoring concepts involve goal setting and clear communication. Formal mentoring, moving through phases and including key tasks and processes, has been outlined (Zachary, 2005). They include an initial selection process for a good mentor-mentee match. Phases such as orienting, working, and disengaging are common. Both mentors and mentees take active roles in the process. Reflection is also considered a central concept of mentoring, with mentor and mentee reflecting together on goals for the relationship, on milestones reached, or on products developed.

As faculty's careers progress, they will adapt a broader mentor role. Not only is this an opportunity to feel positive about their contributions to others, but also a way to pass on knowledge and tips that others have shared with them.

Mentoring Toolkits

A tool for guidance on the mentoring process is the NLN's (2008b) "The Mentoring of Nursing Faculty Toolkit," focused to enhance faculty career development as well as promote healthy work environments. This document describes mentoring programs as early, mid-, and late career programs. A series of questions are provided to guide mentoring assessments and practices at varied career points. Resources are provided to support these relationships.

Mentoring also relates to terms such as coaching and precepting. These terms have some differences but relate basically to guidance and support of less-experienced individuals. For example, the term *coaching* typically relates to short-term relationships rather than extended, goal-directed career activities. A handbook on coaching in nursing has been developed by Sigma Theta Tau and provides many useful tools for mentors to use (Donner & Wheeler, 2009). Other disciplines provide guidance in mentoring as well. For example, Kashiwagi, Varkey, and Cook (2013) completed a literature synthesis of mentoring programs in academic medicine, describing diverse models including dyad, functional, and group approaches to support mentees into a professional culture.

With wide use of the Internet, mentoring is often provided at a distance. Communication and exchange principles are similar, but new approaches using technologies serve to promote student, colleague, and faculty mentoring communications.

Mentoring has many positive outcomes. These include contributions such as meaningful support, sense of belonging, and successful contribution to growth and a career trajectory (Smith, Hecker-Fernandes, Zorn, & Duffy, 2012). Research by Chung and Kowalski (2012) found variables of job satisfaction, quality, stress, and psychological empowerment showed significant positive correlations to mentoring roles. The value of mentoring to the profession as a whole has also been described (Shinn, 2013).

ENGAGE IN SELF-REFLECTION TO IMPROVE TEACHING PRACTICES

Self-reflection as individuals advance through their career trajectory keeps the nurse educator focused on the most important aspect of the life of an educator—that of improving teaching practices. Just as career advancement for a nurse in clinical practice is all about improving patient outcomes, so too is career advancement for a nurse educator all about improving teaching and learning.

Careers are often centered on building experiences and dealing with change and transition. Enhancing a career through these events involves understanding the academic culture and expected facets of a college career. This is a culture that broadly appreciates a focus on documenting progress in education, service, and scholarship activities. The CV and portfolio provide documentation opportunities.

Theories, Evidence, and Tools

Transitions, change, and ongoing quality improvement relate to nursing career planning. CVs and portfolios gain direction from the scholarship of teaching and learning (Boyer, 1990) and resources such as *Making Teaching and Learning Visible* (Bernstein, Burnett, Goodburn, & Savory, 2006). These resources both identify the importance of and provide guidance in naming what is comprised in the professional educator role. Naming what educators do as part of the profession was described as important decades ago by nurse leaders such as Styles (1982). She shared that professions and professionals should conceptualize components of their practice to include naming their products. She further relates naming professional products by incorporating use of best practices and resources. Selected tools and approaches to guide progression, change, and transitions include seeking a good academic fit with documentation via a CV and portfolio.

Seek a Good Academic Fit

Gaining clarity on a particular school's academic system provides a good start for matching personal interests with career planning (Penn et al., 2008). Seek a good academic fit and faculty appointment type that fits with your career goals. This involves knowing about the types of academic settings and types of faculty appointments as well as the concepts of tenure and promotion. Ask questions such as: Will I be adjunct faculty, clinical faculty, or research faculty? Will my role be in a research intensive or a teaching intensive university?

Schools with a specific research mission often require different faculty competencies or processes than those for faculty who want to focus on teaching and service (Bartels, 2007). Research intensive institutions focus more on research products while the academic intensive institutions focus more on educational scholarship. Finding a good match with your interests and the institution's needs is key (Adams, 2002).

A good academic fit involves learning about a program's system for promotion and tenure. Begin with questions such as What type of appointment will I have? What type of education is required for different appointments?

Seek orientation to the organization's policies and procedures related to tenure:

1. The process and calendar to be followed
2. The types of documentation needed by the tenure committee
3. The criteria to be used to assess the tenure packet
4. If and how there is a weighting to the types of faculty activities or outcomes (Diamond, 2002).

Plan to learn about faculty development opportunities provided for selected roles. Finally, develop a CV and, typically, a portfolio that flows from and matches your plan.

Developing a Curriculum Vitae and Portfolio

Career progression focuses around setting career goals and building a CV as the semesters and years advance. Understanding a school's mission, job descriptions, and promotion or tenure guidelines will guide your professional development and progression over time.

Your CV may be referred to as an enhanced résumé and provides a detailed summary used to document progression of professional experiences. The CV involves clearly naming and describing to others what you do and your areas of interest (McBride, 2010). This is a professional document that does not include personal or family information. CV components can relate to the traditional teaching, research, and service roles or Boyer's (1990) expanded criteria. Building a CV includes professional areas an individual wants to emphasize and demonstrate progress in selected roles. McBride (2010) describes the value of documenting transitions or advancement from the home stage to the broader health care professional field. Naming products and activities as one progresses from novice to expert in an area shows professional growth.

A portfolio is a collection of writings and documents that summarize an individual's work and experiences. This can be as simple as a notebook documenting accomplishments and showing samples of work. Portfolio development complements a CV and highlights self-directed, lifelong learning. It includes documenting that learning is occurring. Portfolios can showcase the teaching-learning process and outcomes. Benefits of portfolios include helping to document progress in multiple career components (both in clinical and educator contexts) over time. This document also serves as a reminder to an individual to make career plans happen, gives vision for personal mastery, and indicates how these align with an organization's needs.

There are varied approaches for structuring portfolios. Key concepts include communication about and reflection on what you do. For example, naming and describing a course you teach (perhaps sharing a course developed in a clinical specialty area or emerging interest, such as palliative care or informatics), then reflecting on the course successes and challenges. This portfolio component tells the story of your course development and how you shared this professionally with others as part of professional development. As you create your personal portfolio, each component contributes to the whole. Although different career points in time focus on different areas, the complete portfolio shows the big picture of your career.

SUMMARY

Quality improvement in the educator role includes not just staying busy with activities, but also demonstrating products and progression in the various academic roles. Gaining a vision of what an academic career can look like and finding a good academic setting that matches an individual's interests and skills provide a good beginning to role socialization. Assessing one's strengths and desires, seeking education and mentoring opportunities for lifelong learning, seeking and using feedback, and learning to balance the various roles of an academic nurse educator provide a firm basis for ongoing improvement in career and program quality. This ideally leads to a personal career plan that makes a good match within an employment organization.

Practice Test Questions

1. A peer evaluation of a new faculty member identifies challenges within the classroom teaching. Which strategy is the priority for this new faculty?
   A. Completing a self-assessment rubric of a taped teaching session
   B. Participating in an administrative conference about good teaching
   C. Completing coursework on teaching strategies
   D. Summarizing end of semester student evaluations

2. A new faculty member is seeking an opportunity to advance his professional service work. Which activity indicates the faculty member requires additional mentoring about his service plans?
   A. Increases his family nurse practitioner hours in the primary care clinic
   B. Becomes an active member of a university-wide committee
   C. Joins a nursing organization task group in his specialty
   D. Seeks a school of nursing committee appointment

3. Which statement by a faculty member, concerning career balance, would suggest the need for further mentoring?
   A. I am using what I am learning from my evaluation committee work to help develop my new nursing course.
   B. I am working with a physical therapy colleague to write a paper about functional assessment.
   C. Often I use the same project for both a presentation and then a publication.
   D. My personal goal is to submit three manuscripts I will write this month.

4. Which statement from a new faculty member is most indicative of the need for a more reasonable socialization plan?
   A. I am meeting with other course faculty to learn about student clinical expectations.
   B. My understanding of the program is developing as I review handbooks and meet with program staff.
   C. My personal philosophy for this course will guide my plans as I think about how I want this course to go.
   D. I am meeting with clinical agency staff to better understand how they expect me to teach this course

5. The nursing educator is meeting with new nursing students. Which strategy will the faculty use to promote academic honesty?
   A. Review the course calendar for exam deadlines.
   B. Review the syllabus for student academic integrity guidelines.
   C. Require students to purchase antiplagiarism computer devices.
   D. Require students to work as partners for test taking.

6. Which action should be used first for the student who has repeatedly been late to her clinical practicum?
   A. Fail the student
   B. Have the student sign a contract
   C. Place the student on academic suspension
   D. Review the student handbook

7. As you mentor a faculty colleague, which statement indicates the need for further questioning about professional development plans?

A. I am working to gain certification in my clinical specialty.

B. I am putting together a strategic plan based on my self-assessment using the NLN Certified Nurse Educator competencies.

C. I am making plans to enroll in a doctor of nursing practice program that my administrator wants me to complete.

D. I am participating in a college-wide teaching strategies workshop.

8. Which statement from a nurse educator planning to sign a contract for a new position would be a concern?

A. I will be orienting with and learning from others with similar clinical interests and career goals.

B. I am looking forward to learning about the program orientation and how my interests fit with the organization.

C. I feel like my interests are a good match with the organization's mission.

D. I think the type of appointment being offered will be a good match for my interests.

References

Adams, K. A. (2002). What colleges and universities want in new faculty. Retrieved from http://www.aacu.org/pff/pdfs/PFF_Adams.PDF

Altany, A. (2012). Professional faculty development: The necessary fourth leg. Retrieved from http://www.facultyfocus.com/articles/faculty-development/professional-faculty-development-the-necessary-fourth-leg/

American Association of Higher Education (AAHE). (1996). Ethical principles for college and university teaching. Retrieved from http://www.aahea.org/articles/Ethical+Principles.htm

Bailey, G. (1981). *Teacher self-assessment: A means for improving classroom instruction.* Washington, DC: National Education Association.

Bartels, J. (2007). Preparing nursing faculty for baccalaureate level and graduate level nursing programs: Role preparation for the academy. *Journal of Nursing Education, 46*(4), 154–158.

Benner, P. (1984). *From novice to expert: Excellence and power in clinical nursing practice.* Menlo Park, CA: Addison-Wesley.

Benton, S., & Cashin, W. (2009). Student ratings of teaching: A summary of research and literature. The IDEA Center. Retrieved from http://www.theideacenter.org/research-and-papers/idea-papers/50-student-ratings-teaching-summary-research-and-literature

Bernstein, D., Burnett, A., Goodburn, A., & Savory, P. (2006). *Making teaching and learning visible.* Bolton, MA: Anker.

Biddle, B. (1979). *Role theory: Expectations, identities, and behaviors.* New York: Academic Press.

Blake, A., Ashforth, B., Sluss, D., & Saks, A. (2007). Socialization tactics, proactive behavior, and new-comer learning: Integrating socialization models. *Journal of Vocational Behavior, 70*(7), 447–462.

Boehm, H., & Bonnel, W. (2010). The use of peer review in nursing education and clinical practice. *Journal for Nurses in Staff Development, 26*(3), 108–115.

Bolman, L., & Deal, T. (2008). *Reframing organizations: Artistry, choice, and leadership.* San Francisco: Jossey-Bass.

Bonnel, W. (2008). Improving feedback to students in online courses. *Nursing Education Perspectives, 29*(5), 290–294.

Bonnel, W., & Boehm, H. (2011). Faculty practices in providing online course feedback. *Journal of Continuing Nursing Education, 42*(11), 503–509.

Boyer, E. L. (1990). *Scholarship reconsidered: Priorities of the professoriate.* Princeton, NJ: Carnegie Foundation for the Advancement of Teaching.

Cardinal, B. (2013). Service vs. serve-us: What will your legacy be? *Journal of Physical Education, Recreation & Dance, 84*(5), 4–6.

Chung, C. E., & Kowalski, S. (2012). Job stress, mentoring, psychological empowerment, and job satisfaction among nursing faculty. *Journal of Nursing Education, 51*(7), 381–388.

Diamond, R. (2002). *Serving on promotion, tenures, and faculty review committees, a faculty guide.* Bolton, MA: Anker.

Donabedian, A. (1982). *The criteria and standards of quality.* Ann Arbor, MI: Health Administration Press.

Donner, G., & Wheeler, M. (2009). Coaching in nursing. An introduction. Sigma Theta Tau. Retrieved from http://www.nursingsociety.org/Education/ProfessionalDevelopment/Documents/Coaching%20and%20Mentoring%20Workbook_STTI.pdf

Fink, L. (2003). *Creating significant learning experiences: An integrated approach to designing college courses.* San Francisco: Jossey-Bass.

Gaberson, K., & Oermann, M. (2010). *Clinical teaching strategies in nursing* (3rd ed.). New York: Springer.

Glaserfeld, E. (1989). *Constructivism in education.* Oxford, England: Pergamon.

Hiemstra, R. (2010). Techniques, tools, and resources for the self-directed learner. Retrieved from http://www-distance.syr.edu/sdltools.html

Institute of Medicine (IOM). (2003). *Health professions education: A bridge to quality.* Washington, DC: National Academies Press.

Institute of Medicine (IOM). (2011). *The future of nursing: Leading change, advancing health.* Washington, DC: National Academies Press.

Kahanov, L., Eberman, L, Yoder, A., & Kahanov, M. (2012). Culture shock: Transitioning from clinical practice to educator. *Internet Journal of Allied Health Sciences and Practice, 10*(1). Retrieved from http://ijahsp.nova.edu/articles/Vol10Num1/pdf/Kahanov.pdf

Kashiwagi, D., Varkey, P., & Cook, D. (2013). Mentoring programs for physicians in academic medicine: A systematic review. *Academic Medicine, 88*(7), 1029–1037.

Knowles, M., Holton, E. F., & Swanson, R. A. (1998). *The adult learner: The definitive classic in adult education and human resource development* (5th ed.). Houston: Gulf Publishing.

Kurtzman, E., & Johnson, J. (2012). Quality and safety in healthcare: Policy issues. In D. Mason, J. Leavitt, & M. Chaffee (Eds.), *Policy and politics in nursing and healthcare* (pp. 366–374). St. Louis. Elsevier Saunders.

Massey, W., Graham, S., & Short, P. (2007). *Academic quality work: A handbook for improvement.* Bolton, MA: Anker.

McBride, A. (2010). *The growth and development of nurse leaders.* New York: Springer.

McKeachie, W. J., & Svinicki, G. (2013). *McKeachie's teaching tips: Strategies, research, and theory for college and university teachers* (13th ed.). Belmont, CA: Wadsworth.

Myers, J., & Jaeger, J. (2012). Faculty development in quality improvement: Crossing the educational chasm. *American Journal of Medical Quality, 27*(2), 96–97.

National Council of State Boards of Nursing (NCSBN). (2011). White paper: A nurse's guide to the use of social media. Retrieved from https://www.ncsbn.org/Social_Media.pdf

National League for Nursing (NLN). (2006). Healthful work environment toolkit. Retrieved from http://www.nln.org/facultyprograms/HealthfulWorkEnvironment/toolkit.pdf

National League for Nursing (NLN). (2008a). Informatics education toolkit. Retrieved from http://www.nln.org/facultyprograms/facultyresources/index.htm

National League for Nursing (NLN). (2008b). The mentoring of nursing faculty toolkit. Retrieved from http://www.nln.org/facultyprograms/MentoringToolkit/

National League for Nursing (NLN). (2012a). Certified nurse educator candidate handbook, 2012–2013. Retrieved from http://www.nln.org/certification/handbook/cne.pdf

National League for Nursing (NLN). (2012b). The fair testing imperative in nursing education: A living document. Retrieved from http://www.nln.org/aboutnln/livingdocuments/pdf/nlnvision_4.pdf

Penn, B., Wilson, L., & Rosseter, R. (2008). Transitioning from nursing practice to a teaching role. *Online Journal of Issues in Nursing, 13*(3). Retrieved from http://www.nursingworld.org/MainMenuCategories/ANAMarketplace/ANAPeriodicals/OJIN/TableofContents/vol132008/No3Sept08/NursingPracticetoNursingEducation.aspx

Sawatzky, J., & Enns, C. (2009). A mentoring needs assessment: Validating mentorship in nursing education. *Journal of Professional Nursing, 25*(3), 145–150.

Schon, D. (1987). *Educating the reflective practitioner.* San Francisco: Jossey-Bass.

Shinn, L. (2013). Current issues in nursing associations. In D. Mason, J. Leavitt, & M. Chaffee (Eds.), *Policy and politics in nursing and healthcare* (pp. 602–608). St. Louis: Elsevier Saunders.

Slimmer, L. (2012). A teaching mentorship program to facilitate excellence in teaching and learning. *Journal of Professional Nursing, 28*(3), 182–185.

Smith, S., Hecker-Fernandes, J., Zorn, C., & Duffy, L. (2012). Precepting and mentoring needs of nursing faculty and clinical instructors: Fostering career development and community. *Journal of Nursing Education, 51*(9), 497–503.

Styles, M. (1982). *On nursing: Toward a new endowment.* St Louis: CV Mosby.

Tippitt, M., Ard, N., Kline, J., Tilghman, J., Chamberlain, B., & Meagher, G. (2009). Creating environments that foster academic integrity. *Nursing Education Perspectives, 30*(4), 239–244.

Zachary, L. J. (2005). *Creating a mentoring culture. The organization's guide.* San Francisco: Jossey-Bass.

6

Function as a Change Agent and Leader

Theresa M. "Terry" Valiga, EdD, RN, CNE, FAAN, ANEF

The CNE Test Plan Lists the Following for the Area of Function as a Change Agent and Leader:

6. Engage in Scholarship, Service, and Leadership

A. Function as a Change Agent and Leader

1. Function as a change agent and leader
- Model cultural sensitivity when advocating for change
- Evaluate organizational effectiveness in nursing education

2. Enhance the visibility of nursing and its contributions by providing leadership in the:
- nursing program
- parent institution
- local community
- state or region

3. Participate in interdisciplinary efforts to address health care and educational needs:
- within the institution
- locally
- regionally

4. Implement strategies for change within the:
- nursing program
- institution
- local community

5. Develop leadership skills in others to shape and implement change

6. Adapt to changes created by external factors

7. Create a culture for change within the:
- nursing program
- institution

8. Advocate for nursing, nursing education, and higher education in the political arena

The National League for Nursing (NLN) Certification Commission Certification Test Development Committee (2012, p. 19) asserts that "nurse educators function as change agents and leaders to create a preferred future for nursing education and nursing practice." To function effectively as a change agent and leader, the nurse educator:

- Models cultural sensitivity when advocating for change
- Integrates a long-term, innovative, and creative perspective into the nurse educator role
- Participates in interdisciplinary efforts to address health care and educational needs locally, regionally, nationally, or internationally
- Evaluates organizational effectiveness in nursing education
- Implements strategies for organizational change

- Adapts to changes created by external factors
- Provides leadership in the parent institution as well as in the nursing program to enhance the visibility of nursing and its contributions to the academic community
- Promotes innovative practices in educational environments
- Develops leadership skills to shape and implement change
- Advocates for nursing education and higher education in the political arena

It is clear from this charge that taking on the responsibility of leadership and functioning as a change agent in and for nursing education is something that lies within each faculty member and is not limited only to those who hold formal administrative positions in an organization. Too often faculty look to department chairs, program directors, or deans to formulate a vision for program development in a particular school; the reality, however, is that faculty need to be leaders who help articulate and then shape that vision—that preferred future—for the school. Likewise, faculty often look to boards of national organizations to determine standards related to education and feel they have no role in determining what excellence in nursing education looks like. The reality, again, is that faculty need to be the leaders and change agents who define excellence, identify the support and resources needed to achieve excellence, and lead change initiatives designed to continually pursue that goal. Leadership, therefore, is not something that belongs only to individuals in formal positions of authority. But what is leadership? And how is it the same as, and different from, management?

FUNCTION AS A CHANGE AGENT AND LEADER; ENHANCE THE VISIBILITY OF NURSING AND ITS CONTRIBUTIONS BY PROVIDING LEADERSHIP

Grossman and Valiga (2013, p. 1) acknowledge that "defining just what leadership is, who leaders are, what leaders do, and how leadership is different from management—a phenomenon with which it often is confused—is no easy task." These authors assert that leadership and management are different, leadership can be learned, and each of us can and should be a leader; these concepts are congruent with the competency the NLN has outlined for nurse educators.

Management is a function carried out by individuals in formal positions of authority. By virtue of their position, such individuals are expected to ensure their subordinates work to fulfill the goals of the organization, often have an eye on the "bottom line" rather than on the horizon, and work to minimize disruption so tasks can be accomplished. Their power comes from their position and may be demonstrated through reward and punishment.

Conversely, leadership is a function carried out by any number of individuals in an organization. Leaders have their eye on a long-term vision of excellence, a vision they articulate clearly and with passion, and which serves to entice others to join efforts to achieve it. Leaders, therefore, arise from the group and are given power to influence that group by virtue of their knowledge, credibility, passion, and ability to motivate others. They work collaboratively with followers to achieve a goal that is created and shared by all and not merely imposed by the organization.

Leaders and Followers

Many often bristle at the notion of themselves or others being thought of as followers. In essence, however, there can be no leaders if there are no followers. But effective followers are not sheep who follow blindly. Instead, they are thinking, passionate, motivated individuals who participate actively in making change happen and shaping a new, preferred future.

Essentially, effective followers have many of the same characteristics as leaders. They are forward-looking, question and challenge the status quo, are comfortable with change, are willing to take risks, are actively involved, and think critically about and challenge ideas that are presented to determine the best possible decision or course of action.

Followers with these characteristics often assume a leadership role when needed to keep the group moving toward its vision, and they build positive, reciprocal relationships with the entire team, including the identified leader. Followers, therefore, are critical for change to occur, and they are essential if leaders are to help shape a preferred future.

Managers and Administrators as Leaders

As noted, every faculty member has the opportunity—and the responsibility—to take on the role of leader when needed to continually improve nursing education. And many faculty do take on this responsibility. But leadership in an organization is also provided by faculty who hold positions such as course coordinators, level coordinators, or committee chairs, as well as by individuals who are in formal positions of authority—deans, chairpersons, directors, and so on.

Leaders, as previously noted, often emerge from and are followed by members of a group because of the vision they espouse. Individuals in formal positions of authority, on the other hand, typically are appointed by some external individual or group (e.g., vice president for academic affairs, provost). Such appointments, however, reflect support of the individual's vision for the school or program, ability to help a group or organization grow and evolve, and ability to lead change. Thus, they have many of the same characteristics that have been described for leaders.

Deans and directors are expected to collaborate with faculty to outline goals for the school or program and formulate plans to reach those goals. Such goals might include increasing the number of qualified applicants, increasing graduation rates, improving program outcomes, offering programs in online or hybrid formats, increasing the number of doctorally prepared faculty, increasing the amount of external grant funds received, offering new graduate-level specialties, or enhancing the influence of the school or program within the parent institution. These are examples of important goals that require extensive planning and resources to achieve and are met through collaborative efforts among administrators, faculty, clinical partners, and other offices or departments within the institution.

Administrators have the responsibility for ensuring the work of the school or program is aligned with that of the parent institution, and often they are called upon to provide evidence of such congruence. They have overall responsibility for developing and managing the budget for the school or program, often are the final decision-makers related to faculty appointments, and are expected to provide input to committees or higher-level administrators regarding faculty promotion or tenure decisions.

Faculty who aspire to an administrative role, therefore, need to develop strong management skills as well as skills of leadership. They need to learn to effectively balance those responsibilities. The dean or director who puts too much emphasis on management may contribute to the evolution of a highly efficient system with a "positive bottom line," but one with a system that is unwilling to change for fear of introducing uncertainties, raising the possibility of failure, and jeopardizing efficient operations. On the other hand, the dean or director who puts too much emphasis on leadership may contribute to the evolution of a system that is in constant flux, does not stay within its budget, has no clear sense of direction, and does not meet expectations set by upper administration. It is important, therefore, that individuals in formal positions of authority know when to "push" change and innovation and when to move toward change in a cautious, deliberate manner.

IMPLEMENT STRATEGIES FOR CHANGE; DEVELOP LEADERSHIP SKILLS IN OTHERS TO SHAPE AND IMPLEMENT CHANGE

As noted previously, both leaders and followers are driven toward excellence and a preferred future, and administrators or managers typically value excellence as well. To reach such goals, it must be understood that change is essential and that members of the organization are challenged to think in new ways and are supported as they encounter the uncertainties on that journey. All administrators and faculty understand that change is a "messy" process. Although experts have outlined phases of change that may suggest all that is needed is to follow that path and all will be well, the truth is that change can be quite threatening to many individuals. Feeling threatened may prompt individuals to act in ways that seem to "stall" or provide "roadblocks" to achieve the new goal.

The effective leader and change agent recognizes that attention must be paid to the individuals in the group—their backgrounds, past experiences with change, self-confidence, comfort with ambiguity and uncertainty, cultural practices, and sense of vulnerability (e.g., are they approaching a tenure or promotion review and unwilling to openly oppose ideas presented by members of the committee that will review their dossier?). Attention must also be paid to the group as a whole, taking into consideration the group's past experiences with change and its aftermath, the degree of collegiality and civility (Clark, 2013) in the group, the group's culture regarding decision-making, and the resources available to support change efforts.

Motivating and leading a group to change involve the stages outlined by Lewin (1951). Although this theory was proposed more than 60 years ago, it still has relevance and is still useful to leaders. Lewin noted the first phase of change is that of *unfreezing*, during which members of the group prepare for change. Once the need for change has been accepted, the phase of *moving* occurs where the design and implementation of the change itself takes place. Finally, the phase of *refreezing* occurs as the change is integrated into the system and becomes part of the new norm.

The perspective on change suggested by Lewin (1951) is one of evolution; a change is planned, gradually introduced, and may take an extended period of time before it becomes fully integrated into the system and culture of the organization or group. Conversely, recent literature (Christensen, Baumann, Ruggles, & Sadtler, 2006) addresses a more revolutionary perspective on change. Disruptive innovations or technologies serve to turn systems upside down rather quickly, ideas are adopted rapidly, and groups or organizations strive to be "on the cutting edge" in the field. Such change may be referred to as transformative, in which the *structure* of organizations (i.e., who reports to whom, the names and functions of departments or subunits), the *processes* within organizations (i.e., how decisions are made), and the *culture* of organizations or groups (i.e., how things are viewed, what is valued and rewarded) are dramatically changed.

The nursing education leader needs to be comfortable with both evolutionary and revolutionary change. For example, when proposing a new curriculum that eliminates specialty silos, focuses on integration, is open and flexible, attends more to competency than to "seat time," and engages teachers and students as colearners, faculty colleagues may need extended time to prepare for and implement such a change. The leader might circulate articles or books that address the need to transform nursing education (and health professions education in general), negotiate with administrators to bring experts to the school to talk about their experiences with creating and implementing such curricula, provide extensive opportunities for dialogue and expression of concern about the change, and outline a clear timeline of the steps that need to be taken to achieve the goal in a reasonable timeframe.

Conversely, faculty who are early adopters of various technologies and appreciate the need to fully integrate technology into the educational program may promote a more revolutionary approach to change. They may gather together to form a group to pilot various technologies, document the outcomes of those "experiments," make revisions based on the outcomes, report findings to the larger faculty, encourage and mentor others to try new approaches in their courses, and continue to move ahead with integrating the technology even if everyone else is not "on board."

Whichever approach to change is used, the leader must take the risk of offering new ideas or approaches, influencing others to "get on board," and collaborate with followers to sustain the change. This influence is needed within the school or program, but it also is needed on a broad level as well.

PARTICIPATE IN INTERDISCIPLINARY EFFORTS; ADAPT TO CHANGES CREATED BY EXTERNAL FACTORS; CREATE A CULTURE FOR CHANGE; ADVOCATE FOR NURSING AND EDUCATION IN THE POLITICAL ARENA

Effective nursing education leaders have a broad perspective, are not limited in their thinking, are aware of external forces that impact nursing education, learn from colleagues in other fields, and work to create a preferred future within their own program, the larger institution, the community, and the field in general. They serve on institutional committees that address educational standards, outcomes assessment, educational technology, student engagement, or ongoing development of the pedagogical expertise of faculty. They read the educational literature and follow education-focused listservs, while keeping current in the clinical areas they teach. They attend conferences related to nursing and health professions education, educational technology, and issues in higher education, and they participate in national organizations that focus on shaping nursing and higher education.

Nursing education leaders also initiate discussions of appointment, promotion, and tenure criteria to heighten awareness of the need to recognize and reward excellence and innovation in teaching, leadership in curriculum development, and the scholarship of teaching and learning, not just the traditional activities of research, grant funding, and peer-reviewed publications. Such discussions can take place within one's school, one's institution, or at the regional and national levels. Does action such as this involve risk? Indeed, it does. But, as noted earlier, leaders are risk takers who often say what needs to be said and challenge traditional ways of thinking and the status quo.

In addition to these activities, nursing education leaders are involved politically. They advocate for funding to support educational innovations, faculty development, and pedagogical research. They meet with legislators—in the local community, at the state level, or at the national level—to educate political figures about the nature of our work as educators, the focus of nursing education, the significance and challenges of clinical learning experiences, and the need for evidence-based teaching practices, among other issues. Some also may assume roles as political leaders to ensure they are "at the table" and in a position to bring the wisdom, insights, and perspectives of nurse educators to significant issues under discussion.

Finally, it also is important that nursing education leaders serve as mentors to others who desire to shape a preferred future for the field. Providing opportunities for faculty colleagues to colead change efforts, "experiment" with new approaches to teaching or learning, or develop proposals for a new committee structure, advisement system, or revised curriculum is one way a leader can mentor others. The leader also can encourage colleagues who share the passion for educational innovation to become involved in organizations that shape the field at the national level. Additionally, the leader can mentor other faculty by inviting them to coauthor publications or copresent papers at conferences.

SUMMARY

It should be clear from this discussion that nursing education leaders look outward, not inward. They envision new ways to approach nursing education, to implement the faculty role, or to engage students actively in the learning process. They express this vision clearly and with passion. They work with followers—individuals who also support the vision—and with key stakeholders (e.g., students, faculty from other disciplines, administrators, legislators) to design and implement the changes needed to realize the vision. And they are rewarded when excellence is defined and achieved.

Every faculty member needs to think of her- or himself as a leader and not abdicate that responsibility to the dean, program director, or department chairperson. Nursing faculty are role models for students and prepare students to be leaders in nursing. Faculty must be willing to take the risk of trying new things and new ways of doing.

Practice Test Questions

1. Which explanation highlights the differences between leaders and managers?
   A. Leaders focus on task accomplishment; mangers focus on long-term goals.
   B. Leaders' power comes from their role in the organization; managers' power comes from their knowledge.
   C. Leaders' goals arise from a passion for excellence; mangers' goals arise from those of the organization.
   D. Leaders direct subordinates in their work; managers collaborate with followers.

2. What action is best for the nurse educator leader to effectively role model cultural sensitivity when advocating for change?
   A. Invites all members of the faculty to respond to a survey about the need for the change
   B. Acknowledges that the background and unique perspectives of each member influence how each will react to a proposed change
   C. Asks representatives from various faculty "subgroups" (e.g., tenured or nontenured, educated in or outside the United States) to review a proposed change prior to presenting it to the full faculty
   D. Attends lectures about diversity and cultural differences

3. Which action would be most effective in helping the nursing education leader evaluate the readiness of her or his colleagues for transformative change in the curriculum?
   A. Review the evaluations completed by faculty who attended a presentation on curriculum development
   B. Determine the nature and extent of change experienced by the group in recent years and the support provided by administration for the change
   C. Reflect on the extent to which comments made at a meeting are congruent with her or his own goals
   D. Interview faculty regarding their nursing practice experiences

4. The nurse educator reflects on recent higher education literature about empowering students and envisions a prelicensure program that gives students some choice regarding the assignments they complete for a course and the percentage each will count toward the course grade. By doing this, what is the nurse educator helping to shape?
   A. New workload calculation practices
   B. Collaborative relationships with clinical partners
   C. A preferred future for nursing education
   D. Standards for program evaluation

5. Based on characteristics that describe effective leaders, which action will the nurse educator use to facilitate change and innovation?
   A. Clearly articulate a vision and motivates others to help realize that vision
   B. Seek a position of authority in an organization and is tenured
   C. Chair an important committee in the school and hold the rank of professor
   D. Provide clear instructions to others in completing tasks and set a prescribed timeline for implementation

(continued on page 110)

6. Effective followers display which set of characteristics?
   A. Keep focused on the present; ensure that policies are implemented as prescribed
   B. Challenge new ideas; support members of the group who advocate maintaining the status quo
   C. Accept tasks assigned by the leader without question; listen to all discussions about the new initiative
   D. Collaborate with the leader to design activities to meet the goal; think critically

7. Which responsibility may be assumed by the nurse leader who is *not* in a formal position of authority (i.e., dean, chair, etc.) in the school?
   A. Lead strategic planning efforts for the school as a whole
   B. Develop and oversee implementation of the school's budget
   C. Help members of the faculty engage in evidence-based teaching practices
   D. Serve as a spokesperson for the school within the parent institution

8. Which action by the nurse educator best demonstrates the role of leader and change agent?
   A. Accepting an invitation to run for office in a national organization
   B. Continuing to work in the intensive care unit at least one weekend per month
   C. Advocating to retain the curriculum plan, citing no major negative outcomes of it
   D. Informing students of the benefits of scholarly work

9. Which action by the nurse educator would best demonstrate leadership and enhance the visibility of nursing in the parent institution?
   A. Serving as chair of the school's student affairs committee
   B. Volunteering at a local indigent care clinic
   C. Attending the institution's faculty senate meetings
   D. Coordinating a health fair for faculty and staff of the parent institution

10. First-time pass rates on the licensing exam at the school have been below the national average for the past two years, and the newly appointed chair believes curriculum revision is necessary to address this situation. Drawing on his knowledge of Lewin's change theory, what is the most likely problem this new chair will encounter as he begins to advocate for curriculum change?
   A. Policies that prevent new approaches during the data-gathering stage
   B. Resistance during the unfreezing stage
   C. Sabotage during the refreezing stage
   D. Lack of financial support during the moving stage

References

Christensen, C. M., Baumann, H., Ruggles, R., & Sadtler, T. M. (2006). Disruptive innovation for social change. *Harvard Business Review, 84*(12), 94–101.

Clark, C. (2013). *Creating & sustaining civility in nursing education.* Indianapolis: Sigma Theta Tau International Honor Society of Nursing.

Grossman, S. C., & Valiga, T. M. (2013). *The new leadership challenge: Creating the future of nursing* (4th ed.). Philadelphia: F.A. Davis.

Lewin, K. (1951). *Field theory in social science: Selected theoretical papers.* New York: Harper & Row.

National League for Nursing Certification Commission Certification Test Development Committee. (2012). *The scope of practice for academic nurse educators* (2012 revision). New York: National League for Nursing.

Engage in Scholarship of Teaching

Marilyn Frenn, PhD, RN, CNE, FTOS, ANEF

The CNE Test Plan Lists the Following for the Area of Engage in Scholarship of Teaching:

6. Engage in Scholarship, Service, and Leadership
 B. Engage in Scholarship of Teaching
  1. Exhibit a spirit of inquiry about teaching and learning, student development, and evaluation methods
  2. Use evidence-based resources to improve and support teaching
  3. Participate in research activities related to nursing education
  4. Share teaching expertise with colleagues and others
  5. Demonstrate integrity as a scholar

The task statements noted in the detailed Certified Nurse Educator (CNE) test blueprint for Category 6B reflect the nurse educator's role related to the scholarship of teaching. As noted, there are five major areas covered in this section, each equally important to the scholarship of teaching.

EXHIBIT A SPIRIT OF INQUIRY ABOUT TEACHING AND LEARNING, STUDENT DEVELOPMENT, AND EVALUATION METHODS

A spirit of inquiry is within the nature of a scholar. A scholar is a member of a profession who is able to think logically and is a self-directed thinker. The scholar is able to develop new ideas and approaches in an attempt to solve problems of the profession. An important element of a scholar is engaging in lifelong learning about an area of expertise. Although knowledgeable about all areas of nursing education, any single faculty member cannot be an expert in all areas. Therefore, a scholar identifies an area of personal interest and engages in scholarly activities related to that interest (Adams & Valiga, 2009; Cannon & Boswell, 2012; Shultz, 2009). The National League for Nursing (NLN) provides a comprehensive overview of the science of nursing education, which provides a foundation for evidence-based teaching and learning in nursing education (Shultz, 2009).

Boyer's (1990) four dimensions of scholarship are an important foundation for understanding perspectives on the nature of inquiry. He described discovery, integration, application, and teaching as the dimensions of scholarship in higher education.

Discovery is associated with epistemologies most commonly known as research. Boyer (1990, p. 17) described this dimension of inquiry as "demonstrating palpable excitement in the life of the institution." The National League for Nursing (NLN,

2012b, 2012c) convened a think tank on nursing education research priorities and has since promulgated a vision for transforming research in nursing education and priorities for this research. The NLN has funded nursing education research for more than a decade.

The scholarship of integration is a process of pulling together isolated facts in a meaningful way to generate new insights. Building bridges across disciplinary knowledge is an example Boyer (1990) gave where insights might be generated in this dimension. The notion of scholarship incorporates the idea that the work is judged as meritorious by worthy peers. Ward (2008) provided a rubric for evaluation of scholarly integration work and other aspects of Boyer's conceptualization of scholarship that might not be published. This was developed to help faculty understand various types of scholarship and improve the quality of work through peer review.

The scholarship of application is putting knowledge to use in addressing consequential problems (Boyer, 1990). Rather than doing social good or being a good citizen per se, scholarship of application requires action flowing from faculty members' expertise (Billings & Halstead, 2012). The action in turn informs their body of knowledge and accumulated expertise. Eddy (2007) provided examples of evaluation research using specific standards to meet the criteria of scholarship—making a difference in the real world. For example, through rigorous evaluation of programs and curricula, faculty can contribute to knowledge development while improving nursing education.

Teaching itself is the final dimension of scholarship (Boyer, 1990), flowing from Aristotle's view that teaching is the highest form of understanding. Scholarly teaching transforms knowledge, extending it through students who are critical and creative thinkers long after the learning occurred. Allen and Field (2005) differentiated the scholarship of teaching from scholarly teaching. They described systematic inquiry, not usually considered research, but which examined the dynamics of educational interventions that resulted in student learning, and encouraged inquiry beyond individual courses to curricula and disciplinary issues. Corry and Timmins's (2009) teaching portfolio is an example of scholarly teaching. The portfolio included a statement of teaching philosophy, a collection of ways in which evidence was applied to improve student learning, and reflection on these data to elucidate knowledge.

Halstead (2007) reviewed literature on the scholarship of teaching, critiquing Boyer's (1990) approach as possibly too narrow for nursing education. Alternate conceptualizations included modifications of Boyer's model to include knowing, teaching, practice, and service (Riley, Beal, Levi, & McCausland, 2002); theoretical scholarship, clinical scholarship, and research scholarship (Roberts & Turnbull, 1995); and evidence that nursing faculty role behaviors were characterized by discovery and dissemination of knowledge scholarship and teaching scholarship (Naddy, 1994).

More recently Farmer and Frenn (2009) and Lerret and Frenn (2011) used a grounded theory approach to describe characteristics of excellent teachers from the educator's and student's perspectives. Faculty described excellent teachers as those who are current and knowledgeable, clearly deliver the content, and engage in student-centered teaching, thereby drawing students into active learning. Those faculty who knew and honored their students, were enthused about their work, knowledgeable, and student-centered were described as excellent teachers by doctoral students, all of whom had experienced many types of nursing education programs. Brykczynski (2012) reported action research within a narrative pedagogical approach to course revision as an exemplar of the scholarship of teaching. Using research strategies enabled a more reasoned approach to analyze student feedback, refine clinically relevant assignments, with improved student evaluations of the course.

Beyond having a spirit of inquiry only about teaching and learning, the CNE examination blueprint, based on the "Nurse Educator Competencies" (Halstead, 2007), indicates that nursing education scholarship also focuses on student development and evaluation methods, both of which are covered in other chapters of this book. Nursing education scholarship increasingly needs to address student development and evaluation related to interprofessional education (IPE). The Institute of Medicine (2010) reported on the future of nursing that called for IPE wherein students from different disciplines learn together. The Interprofessional Education Collaborative (2011) released core competencies, including role and responsibility development, interprofessional communication, and team building to improve client outcomes. To actualize these efforts, the NLN (2012a) convened a think tank on simulation for IPE to identify best practices, determine opportunities to create relationships that foster IPE, and determine research questions that need to be addressed. The NLN (2012b) nursing education research priorities incorporate requisites for IPE as well as nursing-specific educational inquiry.

USE EVIDENCED-BASED RESOURCES TO IMPROVE AND SUPPORT TEACHING

The second aspect to be reviewed in preparation for the CNE examination relates to the use of evidence-based resources to improve and support teaching. According to Ferguson and Day (2005), evidence-based teaching includes seeking the best evidence for teaching and curricular decisions, considering the needs of students, the faculty member's judgment, and the costs involved. They noted that some evidence is available, but often faculty members use tradition or expert opinion, rather than systematically examined approaches. Emerson and Records (2008, p. 361) further described evidence-based teaching as "the validation, generation, application, and perpetuation of those methods that facilitate the preparation of skilled and thoughtful nurses who function in a constantly evolving, global health care environment."

Oermann (2009) noted issues with the evidence base per se in nursing education. Studies often lack rigor, have small sample sizes, and have not been replicated across settings. Although there are many qualitative and descriptive studies, researchers have not defined concepts or operationalized them in the same manner across studies. Often instruments lack satisfactory estimates of reliability and validity. Randomized controlled studies to compare educational interventions are needed. Better funding for nursing education research is much needed. Meanwhile, collaborative studies across educational institutions, replication using the same instruments, and dissemination of curricular evaluation findings could help. Oermann pointed out that often the evidence is not consulted; innovations are developed but not evaluated. The conduct and dissemination of rigorous systematic reviews using established criteria (e.g., as proposed by Im & Chang, 2012; Morin, 2012; Whittemore & Knafl, 2005) may make evidence more available for use.

In a phenomenological study, six faculty members reported barriers to evidence-based nursing education were lack of time, administrative support, and knowledge of pedagogy (Shenefield, 2012). Although the factors sustaining evidence-based teaching have not been examined, related research may well be considered. Melnyk, Fineout-Overholt, Gallagher-Ford, and Kaplan (2012) noted factors that improved evidence-based practice (EBP) were strong beliefs that EBP improves outcomes, knowledge and skills, mentors, and organizational cultures that support evidence-based action. Because nursing faculty members are largely masters and doctorally prepared (NLN, 2013), the assumption may be made that they possess knowledge and skills for appraisal of evidence. Questions to be considered are whether there is strong belief that evidence improves educational outcomes or whether mentors and organizational cultures support evidence-based nursing education. Faculty members may need to examine their skills for changing individual perspectives and organizational cultures to support evidence-based nursing education.

Similar to evidence-based practice, frameworks have been proposed for evidence-based nursing education. Emerson and Records (2008) proposed the Student, Teaching technique, Comparison, and Outcome format. Cannon and Boswell (2012) reviewed models of evidence-based practice and proposed a format for evidence-based nursing education, including Population (i.e., students, administrators, faculty, alumni, candidates, preceptors, or others), Strategy, Comparison, Outcome, and Time period when applicable.

A first step when appraising research for evidence-based nursing education is clearly stating the question. What teaching-learning practice, curricular innovation, or student development issue requires evidence for decision-making? Databases such as the Cumulative Index for Nursing and Allied Health, Dissertation Abstracts, PubMed, PsychINFO, Educational Resources Information Center, and Cochrane, along with the help of a skilled reference librarian are essential for locating studies. Careful decision-making is needed about years to include, search words to use, and the quality of studies or other manuscripts. Search the reference lists for additionally relevant studies, and use the database functions to examine articles citing the most useful studies and studies similar to those. Often authors use different terminology than a researcher would use when conducting a search, so finding one relevant study can lead to others.

An evidence table is helpful for organizing results of a literature search. A number of evidence rating systems are available, but Ebell et al. (2004) proposed rating the quality of various types of evidence for use with patients. Similar criteria could be applied to nursing education:

A. Recommendation based on consistent and good-quality nursing education evidence.
B. Recommendation based on inconsistent or limited-quality nursing education evidence.
C. Recommendation based on consensus, usual practice, opinion, or case report.

Table 7.1 presents an example of a nursing education evidence table. It is important to note in the table the research question, the databases searched, the citations, subjects (i.e., type of students, demographics), method, results, whether the study was applicable (to the setting, students, faculty, other stakeholders, congruent with laws, accreditation standards, organizational mission, and ethical standards), your rating of the quality of the evidence in that study, and any information on the cost to implement the findings in the educational setting. The bottom of the table provides a space to state recommendations based on all the studies and to rate the quality of the overall evidence leading to the recommendation. If there are many

Table 7.1

Evidence-Based Nursing Education Appraisal

What is your specific teaching-learning, curriculum, student progress question?								
What keywords, databases, years will be searched?								
Citation	Subjects	Method	Measures	Results	Applicable	Strength of Evidence		Cost?
Recommendation:								
Strength of *overall* evidence:								

studies, a better approach might be to prepare a final table with only the studies of good quality that are pertinent and applicable.

When a more extensive review of elements is needed to appraise individual nursing education studies, research texts (e.g., Polit & Beck, 2011) can be consulted. Boxes 7.1 and 7.2 present a quick review of the elements to consider when appraising qualitative and quantitative nursing education research. The Joanna Briggs Institute (http://www.joannabriggs.edu.au) also provides a process and electronic tools for appraisal and synthesis of health-related evidence.

Recent studies provide helpful examples of the application of evidence in nursing education. Oermann (2011) used the best evidence on skill development and retention to develop and test the efficacy of cardiopulmonary resuscitation skills in nursing students. Adamson and Kardong-Edgren (2012) provided a very complete description of issues and approaches for instrument reliability. Related to the development of IPE, Johannsen et al. (2012) exemplified an approach to evidence-based teaching wherein the theoretical foundations of constructivism, meaningful learning, and self-efficacy were applied to give students an opportunity to use prior learning to better understand the professional knowledge of students from another discipline.

BOX 7.1 Elements for Consideration in Appraising Qualitative Nursing Education Research

Is the design appropriate for the research question(s)?

Was a thorough, in-depth, intensive examination of the study aims conducted?

Were the rights of study participants protected, including review by an institutional review board?

Did the sample provide rich data with sufficient time spent to yield saturation of categories?

Was the qualitative method consistently and rigorously applied with sufficient reflexivity to prevent bias?

Do the themes appear to parsimoniously capture the meaning of the narratives?

Does the report give you a clear and meaningful picture of the world of study participants?

> **BOX 7.2 Elements for Consideration in Appraising Quantitative Nursing Education Research**
>
> Were the sample size and selection criteria sufficient for statistical power?
>   Was the strongest design used as appropriate for the research question?
>   Was a clearly identified conceptual framework used to guide choice of variables and educational interventions?
>   Were reliability and validity estimates for instruments provided and acceptable?
>   Were the rights of study participants protected, including review by an institutional review board?
>   Was fidelity to the intervention (if applicable) ensured and diffusion to the control prevented?
>   Was the timing of the collection of data appropriate?
>   Was adequate masking or blinding used for intervention and control groups?
>   Were the statistics used appropriate for the level of measurement (i.e., nominal, ordinal, interval, or ratio levels)?
>   Were conclusions supported by the data?

PARTICIPATE IN RESEARCH ACTIVITIES RELATED TO NURSING EDUCATION

The third aspect of scholarship of teaching examined in the CNE examination is participation in research activities. Besides conducting individual or collaborative nursing education studies, faculty members can contribute by raising questions about current practices. Oermann (2009) noted that many educational practices are untested. Questions can be used to formulate the basis for a literature search, a systematic review, or a conversation among colleagues that may catalyze development of a symposium or conference session, bringing together those with the greatest expertise on the topic of concern. Questions may also inform evaluations of current practices.

Evaluations require a valid and reliable instrument(s). Faculty can participate in instrument development studies to develop tools for later use. They may participate as subjects or as content experts, contributing to face or content validity indices. Because grades could be used in program, course, or educational innovation evaluation, faculty can advocate for equal interval grade scales. Often grade scales were developed without rationale, and a more useful purpose can be made of the data generated every semester. When nonequal intervals are used, ordinal-level statistics must be used to analyze the data. These statistics are not as commonly used, and the power to predict statistically significant results is diminished when compared with interval-level statistics (Polit & Beck, 2011).

Formal processes can be created to stimulate attention to nursing education research. Nurse educators can create a research brief component to faculty meetings. Faculty can take turns reporting on relevant research for their curriculum or student issues or issues in higher education. When admission and progression policies are discussed, a taskforce can be created to examine relevant studies. Faculty teaching in similar areas can send new study citations and abstracts of interest by e-mail, putting application questions on a future meeting agenda. Senior faculty and administrators can advocate that evidence-based teaching is a component of promotion and tenure requirements. They can also mentor others in evidence-based teaching. All faculty members can share interesting studies by mentioning them to colleagues, perhaps by leaving a copy on the lunchroom table or in other common areas.

Nursing education research requires much greater funding to support larger, multisite studies. Faculty can inform funding agencies and policymakers of this need to ensure quality nursing education. They can also contribute to and commend organizations funding nursing education research. The NLN, Sigma Theta Tau International, and the Midwest Nursing Research Society are a few of the organizations funding dissertation and other nursing education research.

In 2003 the NLN Task Group on Teaching Learning proposed many ways faculty members can help to build the science of nursing education. Central to these approaches are a questioning spirit and critical mind. Developing frameworks for the practice of teaching, databases to organize evidence, and measurable outcomes of nursing education are examples provided by Gresley (2009). Faculty members may also demonstrate skill in proposal writing for initiatives such as research, resources, and program and policy development to build the science of nursing education (Halstead, 2007).

SHARE TEACHING EXPERTISE WITH COLLEAGUES AND OTHERS

The fourth component of Scholarship of Teaching on the CNE examination is sharing teaching expertise with colleagues and others. Skilled teachers incorporate evidence-based nursing education seamlessly. They discern which aspects of the evidence are critical to student success in their program, preparing them for lifelong learning and effective practice. Sharing this wisdom with a variety of audiences constitutes this aspect of engaging in nursing education scholarship (Halstead, 2007).

Expertise can be shared in various ways throughout a nursing education career (Halstead, 2007). Novice educators may engage in coursework to better understand teaching, learning, and curricular initiatives. They bring fresh perspectives to discussions with colleagues about the application of pedagogical theories and research to the preparation of nurses for current practice. Novice educators might try approaches based in the literature, discussing options and outcomes with colleagues. More experienced educators could mentor novice faculty, sharing their emerging synthesis of evidence-based nursing education along with clinical, institutional, and financial realities. Teaching expertise could be recognized through certification as a nurse educator, awards, endowed chairs, and special appointments as the faculty member develops (Adams & Valiga, 2009).

The highest-impact initiatives may involve actualizing teaching expertise in program development and institutional initiatives, such as service learning, first-year seminars, and capstone projects (Hutchings, Huber, & Ciccone, 2011). With this approach, faculty learn from reflecting on how their efforts have worked to improve student outcomes, then share this information with interdisciplinary colleagues, thereby further developing knowledge.

DEMONSTRATE INTEGRITY AS A SCHOLAR

While performing all the aspects of engaging in the scholarship of teaching, demonstrating integrity is essential. Engaging in the scholarship of teaching means that faculty understand what is known, examine it, and discover and create new ways of knowing. The more faculty understand, the greater the obligation as scholars to use this knowledge and skill with the integration of "mind and moral virtue" that is called integrity (Shulman, 2008, p. ix). As a component of the NLN's (n.d.) core values, integrity is defined as "respecting the dignity and moral wholeness of every person without conditions or limitation." Integrity has also been described as the congruence between what we say and how we act (Simons, 1999).

Theories of ethics provide us with guidance for action (Bosek & Savage, 2007). Many institutions of higher learning follow the American Association of University Professors (2009) "Statement on Professional Ethics" (Smith, 2012). This statement includes engaging in intellectual honesty, being a role model of ethical standards, protecting students' academic freedom, maintaining confidentiality and refraining from exploitation or discriminatory behaviors, respecting the inquiry of associates, demonstrating collegiality and responsibility for institutional governance, discriminating between action as an individual and as an institutional representative, and being effective teachers and scholars. Best practice requires that faculty socialize students to professional ethical standards (Smith, 2012), which means nursing faculty incorporate ethics as a nurse and as a faculty member (Cannon & Boswell, 2012).

Although some nonresearch educational inquiries may not require ratification by an institutional review board, because of the power faculty members have over students, it is wise to have the protocol reviewed for the protection of students (Aycock & Currie, 2013; Kragelund, 2013). As a vulnerable population, students must be able to choose to participate or be able to decline participation as research subjects with reasonable alternatives available to them. Engaging a research assistant not involved with the course to collect consent documents and holding him or her until the course is finished can provide additional ensurance that students are able to freely ask questions.

Involving students as subjects or as coinvestigators or mentoring them in their own research studies contributes greatly to the evolution of nursing education science and development of the skills of scholarship. Modeling integrity and ethical comportment in the work of faculty provides a more effective message than any content or value taught. It is always exciting when former students inform us that they are pursuing further education as a result of the time spent in our classes.

Practice Test Questions

1. Which best demonstrates the scholarship of discovery?
   A. Conducts an original research study that results in the identification of new knowledge
   B. Designs learning models that facilitate learner application of previous knowledge
   C. Uses a variety of teaching methods to actively engage learners
   D. Applies evidence in service as an organizational leader

2. Based on Boyer's "Model of Scholarship," which faculty activity fulfills a scholarship of discovery?
   A. Develop a criterion-referenced examination using items written at the application and analysis levels of Bloom's taxonomy
   B. Share expertise on the application of genetics in nursing at a state conference
   C. Evaluate a novice in the nursing college using a self-developed rubric based on educational research
   D. Research the effectiveness of problem-based team case studies in achieving positive learning outcomes in a pathophysiology course

3. A new faculty member would like to better engage in the scholarship of teaching. Which is the best action to initiate?
   A. Run for a faculty senator position
   B. Organize an ethnocentric learning experience
   C. Present the outcomes of a service learning project
   D. Practice as a registered nurse one weekend a month

4. A nurse educator has accepted an appointment as a strategic steering committee member at the National League for Nursing. Which of the scholarship roles is the nursing educator fulfilling?
   A. Application
   B. Integration
   C. Discovery
   D. Teaching

5. To demonstrate the "Scholarship of Application," the nurse educator recognizes that to include the work in a portfolio it must include all of the following *except*:
   A. Evaluations of the work, by those who received the service
   B. Any type of service, such as volunteering at the animal shelter
   C. Project goals that were defined, procedures well planned, and actions recorded
   D. Description of how the work broadened the professor's understanding of the field

6. The nurse educator prepares a dossier to include evidence-based teaching. This includes:
   A. Developing an educational innovation
   B. Conducting a systematic review using established criteria
   C. Teaching the course as it always has been taught
   D. Describing the need for time to review the literature

(continued on page 122)

7. To demonstrate sharing of teaching expertise, a faculty member develops a portfolio including:
A. Course syllabi for the past seven years
B. Educational programs he has attended
C. Transcripts demonstrating coursework related to nursing education
D. Publications related to evaluated teaching innovations

8. A student stated he would not inform a patient about aspects of health care that were incongruent with the student's religious beliefs. The nurse educator provides feedback to the student that client autonomy must be respected. How does the nurse educator assess this behavior?
A. This demonstrates integrity as a scholar, because protecting client autonomy is included in professional nursing ethics.
B. The nurse educator violated the student's rights to free speech by providing this feedback.
C. The faculty member should insist that the student change his religious belief or be removed from the program.
D. Client autonomy must only be respected if the client is being asked to participate in research.

9. The nurse educator wants to include current students in a study she is planning to conduct. Which statement about education research bears on this situation?
A. Because this is part of the faculty role, no review for protection of human subjects is required.
B. The nurse educator must pay students involved in research.
C. The nurse educator hires a research assistant who collects consent documents approved by the institutional review board and does not see the de-identified data until the semester has ended.
D. Because the information collected is so important, all students are informed they must participate.

References

Adams, M. H., & Valiga, T. M. (Eds.). (2009). *Achieving excellence in nursing education.* New York: National League for Nursing.

Adamson, K. A., & Kardong-Edgren, S. (2012). A method and resources for assessing the reliability of simulation evaluation instruments. *Nursing Education Perspectives, 33*(5), 334–339.

Allen M. N., & Field, P. A. (2005). Scholarly teaching and scholarship of teaching: Noting the difference. *International Journal of Nursing Education Scholarship, 2*(1), art. 12.

American Association of University Professors. (2009). Statement on professional ethics. Retrieved from http://www.aaup.org/report/statement-professional-ethics

American Nurses Association. (2010). The code for nurses with interpretive statements. Retrieved from http://www.nursingworld.org/MainMenuCategories/EthicsStandards/CodeofEthicsforNurses

Aycock, D. M., & Currie, E. R. (2013). Minimizing risks for nursing students recruited for health and educational research. *Nurse Educator, 38*(2), 56–60. doi: 10.1097/NNE.0b013e3182829c3a

Billings, D. M., & Halstead, J. A. (2012). *Teaching in nursing: A guide for faculty* (4th ed.). St. Louis: Elsevier Saunders.

Bosek, M. S. D., & Savage, T. A. (2007). *The ethical component of nursing education.* Philadelphia: Lippincott Williams & Wilkins.

Boyer, E. (1990). *Scholarship reconsidered: Priorities for the professoriate.* Princeton, NJ: Carnegie Foundation for the Advancement of Teaching.

Brykczynski, K. A. (2012). Teachers as researchers: A narrative pedagogical approach to transforming a graduate family and health promotion course. *Nursing Education Perspectives, 33*(4), 224–228.

Cannon, S., & Boswell, C. (Eds.). (2012). *Evidence-based teaching in nursing: A foundation for educators.* Sudbury, MA: Jones and Bartlett.

Corry, M., & Timmins, F. (2009). The use of teaching portfolios to promote excellence and scholarship in nurse education. *Nurse Education in Practice, 9*(6), 388–392.

Ebell, M. H., Siswek, J., Weiss, B. D., Woolf, S. H., Susman, J., Ewigman, B., & Bowman, M. (2004). Strength of recommendation taxonomy (SORT): A patient-centered approach to grading evidence in the medical literature. *American Family Physician, 69*, 548–556.

Eddy, L. L. (2007). Evaluation research as academic scholarship. *Nursing Education Perspectives, 28*(2), 77–81.

Emerson, R. J., & Records, K. (2008). Today's challenge, tomorrow's excellence: The practice of evidence-based education. *Journal of Nursing Education, 47*(8), 359–370.

Farmer, B. J., & Frenn, M. (2009). Teaching excellence: What great teachers teach us. *Journal of Professional Nursing, 25*, 267–272.

Ferguson, L., & Day, R. A. (2005). Evidence-based nursing education: Myth or reality? *Journal of Nursing Education, 44*(3), 107–115.

Gresley, R. S. (2009). Building a science of nursing education. In C. M. Schultz (Ed.), *Building a science of nursing education: Foundation for evidence-based teaching-learning* (pp. 1–13). New York: National League for Nursing.

Halstead, J. (2007). *Nurse educator competencies: Creating an evidence-based practice for nurse educators.* New York: National League for Nursing.

Hutchings, P., Huber, M. T., & Ciccone, A. (2011). *The scholarship of teaching and learning reconsidered: Institutional integration and impact.* San Francisco: Jossey-Bass.

Im, E.-O., & Chang, S. J. (2012). A systematic integrated literature review of systematic integrated literature reviews in nursing. *Journal of Nursing Education, 51*, 632–645.

Institute of Medicine. (2010). *The future of nursing: Leading change, advancing health.* Washington, DC: National Academies Press.

Interprofessional Education Collaborative Expert Panel. (2011). *Core competencies for interprofessional collaborative practice: Report of an expert panel.* Washington, DC: Interprofessional Education Collaborative.

Johannsen, A., Bolander-Laksov, K., Bjurshammar, N., Nordgren, B., Fridén, C., & Hagströmer, M. (2012). Enhancing meaningful learning and self-efficacy through collaboration between dental hygienist and physiotherapist students—a scholarship project. *International Journal of Dental Hygiene, 10*, 270–276. doi: 10.1111/j.1601-5037.2011.00539.x

Kragelund, L. (2013). The obser-view: A method of generating data and learning. *Nurse Researcher, 20*(5), 6–10.

Lerret, S., & Frenn, M. (2011). Challenge with care: Reflections on teaching excellence. *Journal of Professional Nursing, 27*, 378–384.

Melnyk, B. M., Fineout-Overholt, E., Gallagher-Ford, L., & Kaplan, L. (2012). The state of evidence-based practice in US nurses: Critical implications for nurse leaders and education. *Journal of Nursing Administration, 42*, 410–417.

Morin, K. (2012). Fostering rigorous critique of the evidence. *Journal of Nursing Education, 51*, 663–664. doi: 10.3928/01484834-20121119–01

Naddy, D. (1994). Applying Boyer's scholarship model to nurse faculty role behaviors. *Dissertation Abstracts International, 55*(6), 2158B.

National League for Nursing (NLN). (n.d.). *About the NLN.* Retrieved from http://www.nln.org/aboutnln/corevalues.htm

National League for Nursing (NLN). (2012a). *A nursing perspective on simulation and interprofessional education (IPE): A report from the National League for Nursing's think tank on using simulation as an enabling strategy for IPE.* Retrieved from www.nln.org/.../pdf/nursing_perspective_sim_education.pdf

National League for Nursing (NLN). (2012b). 2012–2015 NLN research priorities in nursing education. Retrieved from http://www.nln.org/research-grants/priorities.htm

National League for Nursing (NLN). (2012c). NLN vision: Transforming research in nursing education. Retrieved from www.nln.org/aboutnln/livingdocuments/nln_vision.htm

National League for Nursing (NLN). (2013). Highest earned credential of full-time nurse educators by rank, 2009. *NLN DataView™.* Retrieved from www.nln.org/full/url

Oermann, M. H. (2009). Evidenced-based programs and teaching/evaluation methods: Needed to achieve excellence in nursing education. In M. H. Adams & T. M. Valiga (Eds.), *Achieving excellence in nursing education* (pp. 63–76). New York: National League for Nursing.

Oermann, M. H. (2011). Toward evidence-based nursing education: Deliberate practice and motor skill learning. *Journal of Nursing Education, 50,* 63–64. doi: 10.3928/01484834-20110120-01

Polit, D. F., & Beck, C. T. (2011). *Nursing research: Generating and assessing evidence for nursing practice* (9th ed.). Philadelphia: Lippincott Williams & Wilkins.

Riley, J., Beal, J., Levi, P., & McCausland, M. (2002). Revisioning nursing scholarship. *Journal of Nursing Scholarship, 34,* 383–389.

Roberts, K., & Turnbull, B. (1995). Scholarly productivity: Are nurse academics catching up? *Australian Journal of Advanced Nursing, 20,* 8–14.

Shenefield, D. C. (2012). *Faculty perceptions toward the scholarship of teaching.* (Capella University, publication 3544525). ProQuest Dissertations and Theses, 156. Retrieved from http://search.proquest.com/docview/1234067448?accountid=100. (1234067448).

Shulman, L. S. (2008). Forward. In G. E. Walker, C. M. Golde, L. Jones, A. Conkline Bueschel, & P. Hutchings (Eds.), *The formation of scholars: Rethinking doctoral education for the twenty-first century* (p. ix), San Francisco: Jossey-Bass.

Shultz, C. M. (Ed.). (2009). *Building a science of nursing education: Foundation for evidence-based teaching-learning.* New York: National League for Nursing.

Simons, T. L. (1999). Behavioral integrity as a critical ingredient for transformational leadership. *Journal of Organizational Change Management, 12*(2), 89–104.

Smith, M. H. (2012). *The legal, professional, and ethical dimensions of education in nursing.* New York: Springer.

Ward, R. W. (2008). Assessment of unpublished scholarly activity: An informal rubric for evaluating faculty performance. *Journal of Chiropractic Education, 22,* 17–22.

Whittemore, R., & Knafl, K. (2005). The integrative review: Updated methodology. *Journal of Advanced Nursing, 52*(5), 546–553. doi: 10.1111/j.1365–2648.2005.03621.x

8

Function Effectively within the Organizational Environment and the Academic Community

Nancy C. Sharts-Hopko, PhD, RN, CNE, FAAN

The CNE Test Plan Lists the Following for the Area of Function Effectively within the Organizational Environment and the Academic Community:

6. Engage in Scholarship, Service, and Leadership
C. Function Effectively within the Organizational Environment and the Academic Community
1. Identify how social, economic, political, and institutional forces influence nursing and higher education
2. Make decisions based on knowledge of historical and current trends and issues in higher education
3. Integrate the values of respect, collegiality, professionalism, and caring to build an organizational climate that fosters the development of learners and colleagues
4. Consider the goals of the nursing program and the mission of the parent institution when proposing change or managing issues
5. Participate on institutional and departmental committees

The task statements noted in the detailed Certified Nurse Educator test blueprint for Category 6C reflect the nurse educator's role within the academic organization and community. As noted, there are five major areas covered in this section, each equally important to this educator role.

OVERVIEW

Nurses who assume academic positions often find the culture of higher education markedly different from that of health care delivery. The shift involves moving from an environment that values evidence-based practice for optimum and cost-effective patient or population health outcomes to one that is committed to students' growth. Nurse educators often need to interpret professional values and goals to align with faculty in other academic units within the institution and to the institution's administration, as well as incorporate input from outside the nursing unit into nursing education programs. Successful nurse educators are attuned not only to effective design and implementation of programs that promote nursing students' mastery of professional learning objectives, but also to the environment of their academic institution as well as the sociopolitical and economic context of higher education in which it operates. To function effectively in an academic environment, the nurse educator:

- Uses knowledge of history and current trends and issues in higher education as a basis for making recommendations and decisions on educational issues;
- Identifies how social, economic, political, and institutional forces influence higher education in general and nursing education in particular;
- Develops networks, collaborations, and partnerships to enhance nursing's influence within the academic community;
- Determines own professional goals within the context of academic nursing and the mission of the parent institution and nursing program;
- Integrates the values of respect, collegiality, professionalism, and caring to build an organizational climate that fosters the development of students and teachers;
- Incorporates the goals of the nursing program and the mission of the parent institution when proposing changes or managing issues;
- Assumes a leadership role in various levels of institutional governance; and
- Advocates for nursing and nursing education in the political arena (National League for Nursing Certification Commission, 2012, p. 22).

IDENTIFY HOW SOCIAL, ECONOMIC, POLITICAL, AND INSTITUTIONAL FORCES INFLUENCE NURSING AND HIGHER EDUCATION

The beginning of nursing as a profession is attributed to Florence Nightingale, and after she launched the Nightingale Training School at St. Thomas's Hospital in London in 1860, hospital schools of nursing, based more or less closely on her model, proliferated in the United States throughout the late 19th and early 20th centuries. Academic nursing education was introduced at Teachers College of Columbia University in New York City in 1900 when Isobel Hampton Robb and Adelaide Nutting introduced a course of study for nursing teachers in "Hospital Economics" (Baer, 2012). According to Baer, Nutting used her love of uniformity to promote standardization of nursing curricula, teacher training, and ethical practice in contrast to the then-prevalent apprenticeship model of professional education. By 1926, 25 U.S. colleges and universities granted bachelor's degrees in nursing, and nursing instructors could prepare for their educational role at Teachers College, where research by nurses began to emerge (Baer, 2012). Baer reported that academic education of nurses remained relatively rare until the end of World War II, when 70,000 nurses became eligible for the G.I. Bill and could afford to attend college. Today, 47 schools of nursing in the United States grant diplomas while the vast majority of new nursing graduates each year graduate from colleges and universities, with the majority, 60 percent, graduating with an associate's degree (HRSA, 2013; NLNAC, 2013a).

Nurse educators need to be aware of the organizational context in which they teach. Schools of nursing may be freestanding or in health professions' educational institutions in association with health care systems, and as such they may offer diplomas as well as associate's, bachelor's, master's, doctor of nursing practice, or doctor of philosophy degrees. They could also be located in traditional colleges or universities that are broadly classified as associate's, bachelor's, master's, doctoral, or research-intensive institutions (Carnegie Foundation for the Advancement of Teaching, 2013). In addition, institutions can be identified as public, private secular, or private religious; not for profit or proprietary; and virtual (online) or campus based.

Faculty within a given institution are categorized as, for example, having tenure, which is a career-long contract; being on a tenure track, or period of probation after which tenure may or may not be granted; or being contingent, on time-limited renewable contracts. And they may be full time or part time, often termed adjunct. Full-time faculty may be ranked, commonly as instructor, assistant professor, associate professor, or professor. The rank of emeritus is an honor bestowed on retired faculty who are deemed to have served with distinction. Faculty should seek clarity about what their academic contract means in terms of full-time or part-time status. Moreover, in the transition from clinical nursing practice, nurse educators can encounter a wide range of academic expectations about how many months an annual contract covers, how many teaching credits they are required to assume in a year, and how much time they are required to spend at the institution, even within an individual school.

It is a standard in the United States that nurse educators hold a graduate degree in nursing (CCNE, 2013; NLNAC, 2013b). As nursing education has moved into the mainstream of higher education during the 20th century, and particularly with the emergence of doctoral education in nursing starting in the 1930s, the role of nursing faculty has evolved toward greater conformity with that observed in other disciplines, particularly if they seek tenure and promotion through the academic ranks. In practical terms, this means there is likely to be some expectation of service beyond the nursing unit in the institution and in the profession and of some degree of scholarly productivity that entails varying institutional standards for grant writing, research, and publication. Nurse educators need to seek clear guidelines about the expectations in their particular institution for retention in their job, promotion, and tenure, if it applies.

Nurse educators will be well served to understand an institution's mission and heritage as they consider where to teach and then how to thrive in that institution after joining the faculty. It is imperative the faculty member embrace the institution's mission, whether that reflects, for example, a particular student population whom it is committed to serve, a particular set of religious values the institution adheres to and promotes, or a commitment to an extensive program of federally funded research. All institutions must attend to the expectations of various stakeholders or communities of interest, which include students and their families, alumni, sponsoring religious entities, donors, employers, the community, professional organizations, as well as local, state, and national governments. Within a college or university this context may differ slightly across academic units.

In some institutions nurse educators are required to earn a doctoral degree within a specified time, and in others they are expected to have earned a doctorate or even completed a postdoctoral fellowship before applying. In addition, accrediting bodies as well as state boards of nursing have specific requirements regarding nurse educators' educational level and focus, and their clinical experience regarding what they are permitted to teach.

MAKE DECISIONS BASED ON KNOWLEDGE OF HISTORICAL AND CURRENT TRENDS AND ISSUES IN HIGHER EDUCATION

The curriculum committee of the precursor of the National League for Nursing published *A Standard Curriculum for Schools of Nursing* in 1917, offering suggestions on how nursing education could be improved and offering course outlines for a three-year program of study (National League of Nursing Education, 1937). In 1918, in response to a meeting the Rockefeller Foundation called to discuss the promotion of public health and preventive medicine, the foundation financed the Committee for the Study of Nursing Education. The committee's report is best known by the name of the social researcher who served as its secretary, Josephine Goldmark. Recommendations focused on the general nursing curriculum as well as the inclusion of public health, preparation and role of school directors, facilities required for high-quality nursing education, and the desirability of schools of nursing having a relationship with universities (Committee for the Study of Nursing Education, 1923).

A report by the Committee on the Grading of Nursing Schools, initiated by nurse training school superintendents in 1925 to investigate the evaluation of nursing schools, led to the establishment of nursing accreditation by the National League for Nursing Education (Anonymous, 1939). Working under the auspices of the Carnegie Corporation of New York, Esther Lucile Brown directed a 1948 study, *Nursing for the Future,* in which recommendations were made that schools of nursing be nationally accredited, that they be affiliated with universities, and that they have separate school budgets. Moreover, Brown advocated the establishment of two-year collegiate courses in nursing, a proposal that was successfully tested by Mildred Montag (1959) and led to the rapid growth in associate degree programs in community colleges.

Since those earlier times, various reports have influenced the development of nursing education, most recently the 2010 Institute of Medicine (IOM) report *The Future of Nursing: Leading Change, Advancing Health.* Nurse educators are working to implement two specific recommendations about the education of nurses: the percentage of bachelor's degree prepared nurses reach 80 percent by 2020, and the number of doctorally prepared nurses be doubled by that year. Among other entities, the Robert Wood Johnson Foundation is monitoring the implementation of these recommendations through a series of funded studies (Evaluating Innovations in Nursing Education, 2013).

Organizations outside of nursing have a vested interest in the quality of educational programs. Many educational institutions seek comprehensive accreditation from one of five regional accreditation organizations (Council for Higher Education Accreditation, 2013). All organizations that accredit schools, including the professional nursing accrediting bodies and state boards of nursing, are authorized to do so by the U.S. Department of Education (DOE, 2013). There has been considerable discussion in recent years about the accountability of higher education institutions to ensure quality and the ability of recent graduates to meet the expectations of employers. The DOE attempts to ensure quality through the standards and procedures of accreditation, although its effectiveness remains a matter of controversy (Riley, 2011). At the same time, there is continual tension across professional education at the undergraduate level over the appropriate balance of professionally focused or technical curriculum content versus the incorporation of courses intended to prepare college graduates as broadly learned individuals through exposure to a substantive background in the liberal arts and sciences (Delbanco, 2012).

An important part of the context of nursing education is the high cost of higher education. The United States has emerged recently from the most serious economic recession since the Great Depression. At the same time, over the past 20 years the cost of higher education has increased at a rate far steeper than the Consumer Price Index (Anonymous, 2012). Public institutions have experienced reduced support from their states, and students across all types of institutions have had more difficulty accessing sufficient financial assistance. In addition, institutions of higher education have benefited from other sources of public funding, including research grants from various federal and state agencies, all of whose activities have been curtailed in the interest of cutting expenditures, balancing budgets, and reducing the federal budgetary deficit. The implication for nurse educators is that academic institutions continually strive to operate as cost-effectively as possible. Some faculty in public institutions have been required to take furloughs, increase their teaching loads, or accept reductions in salary (Levine & Scorsone, 2011). Private institutions have been affected as endowments and alumni giving have decreased and as students have been more sensitive to comparative educational costs when exploring and applying to schools of nursing.

Nursing education is fortunate in that while the market for nursing graduates tightened up during the recent economic recession, the prospects for the employability of graduates is strong for the longer term as baby boomer–era nurses retire, as more previously uninsured people are enabled to access health care, and as a growing cadre of older adults require health services (Benson, 2013; U.S. Department of Health and Human Services, 2013). As health care in the United States transitions to a system that is more community based and prevention oriented, nurse educators will be challenged to collaborate with health care administrators to design educational programs that prepare graduates for interprofessional practice in nonhospital-centric settings.

Interprofessional education has emerged in recent years as an important strategy for increasing quality and safety in the delivery of health care. The 1999 IOM report *To Err Is Human* alerted the nation to the fact that at least 98,000 people die per year in U.S. hospitals due to medical error, and hundreds of thousands more experience injury. This report was the beginning of numerous initiatives to enhance quality and safety in the delivery of care, to promote evidence-based practice as a strategy leading to better and more cost-effective care, and specifically to focus on the role of communication in health systems in preventing errors. Interprofessional education is intended to promote effective functioning of health care teams by leveling intrateam hierarchies, enhancing communication, and promoting safety for any team member to identify a potential error before it occurs (Larson, 2012). Not all schools of nursing have the opportunity to collaborate with students majoring in other health professions. Yet there may be opportunities to work with faculty in schools of law, business, engineering, or programs in ethics to develop learning or service opportunities that are potentially enriching and meaningful for all student participants.

In addition to greater inclusion of previously uninsured populations and a shift in the locus of care, the historical trend of new recognition of populations with particular issues, such as, currently, veterans returning from the Iraq and Afghan wars, represents a challenge to nurse educators as they prepare students to interact with patients holistically and recognize their unique needs (American Nurses Association, 2013). Additional examples of historical events that provoked nurse educators to re-evaluate how curricula addressed specific population needs include those affected by Hurricane Katrina in 2005 and current international concerns about how the effects of global warming on the environment may affect population health.

One additional trend that bears discussion is the increasing recognition of nurse educators that students must be prepared to consider health globally even if they practice in a geographically restricted area. Throughout their careers students will encounter patients and colleagues from around the world, and many will have opportunities to study or practice in markedly different cultural contexts. Many schools of nursing now offer their students international immersion experiences typically for a period of two or three weeks following a period of classroom preparation and orientation to the site and the culture. In addition to gaining appreciation for the interplay among culture, geography, and health, an additional learning outcome is the ability to compare differing health care delivery systems.

Nursing organizations such as Sigma Theta Tau International (2013) and the International Council of Nurses (2013), of which the American Nurses Association is a member, provide resources to encourage nursing education related to the advancement of promoting health globally. Specific examples of areas of focus include nurses' support for achievement of the Millennium Development Goals and the education of girls, identification of educational competencies for nurses and midwives around the world, monitoring the migration of nurses from developing countries, and promoting safe work environments for nurses. Both organizations maintain affiliation with the World Health Organization.

INTEGRATE THE VALUES OF RESPECT, COLLEGIALITY, PROFESSIONALISM, AND CARING TO BUILD AN ORGANIZATIONAL CLIMATE THAT FOSTERS THE DEVELOPMENT OF LEARNERS AND COLLEAGUES

Academic institutions express the cultural values of respect and collegiality, which date back to the medieval origin of universities. The earliest European universities, such as the University of Paris or Cambridge University, comprised learned clerics who moved in proximity to libraries and offered lectures for which students paid individually. As academic systems coalesced, professors underwent a probationary period—often to determine whether their teaching conformed to Catholic doctrine—after which they were granted tenure, and with that an understanding that they had academic freedom with regard to their content.

In modern times, a dispute at Stanford University between an economics professor and Mrs. Leland Stanford caused American college professors to establish the American Association of University Professors (AAUP) in 1915 with the aim of protecting the academic freedom of faculty and ensuring due process in matters of employment, including tenure (AAUP, 2013). In some institutions, the AAUP chapter is a collective bargaining unit that represents unionized faculty in the development of their contracts. In other institutions it is a membership organization only, but affords faculty access to resources related to academic freedom, tenure, nondiscrimination, and educational quality.

In general, academic freedom refers to faculty members' expertise in regard to their content and self-determination as to the methods by which they teach; their freedom to determine their topic and methods of research in their discipline; and their right to control curricula in their discipline, admission standards for students, and standards for the evaluation of peers for employment, tenure, and promotion. The AAUP acknowledges religious constraints that may have a bearing on the academic freedom of faculty and notes that these need to be identified prior to a faculty member's employment. Additional constraints may be found in proprietary schools in which people are employed for specific instructional roles and in relation to a faculty member's contract in any institution (e.g., if a faculty member is employed specifically to teach a preexisting learning module online). Still, faculty members who fulfill employment criteria are presumed to be expert about their content.

Academic integrity is an issue of enormous importance for nurse educators as teachers and as scholars, and it is related to an ethos of respect. It is imperative for faculty to know their institutions' policies related to academic standards as well as their academic unit's standards related to scholarship. Students' ability to instantaneously access material on the Internet and the longevity of false information increase the challenge faculty face in explaining to students how important it is to trace the origin of ideas and facts that they cite (Szabo & Underwood, 2004). Faculty members need to familiarize themselves with the types of resources that are advertised to students, such as term paper and thesis writing companies. If students seek consultation for writing or statistical analysis, it is important that faculty are clear about the parameters for use of these resources. A recent trend in higher education related to this topic is the accessibility of technological means for cheating, which include miniature cameras and speakers available at low cost online.

Faculty have access to Internet-based tools into which papers can be submitted to determine the percentage of material that is not original, after which the faculty make an evaluation of the report. For example, 10 percent of a well-written paper may be unoriginal, but it may be accounted for by the reference list. The inclusion of quotes that are properly cited will increase the percentage of unoriginal material. In addition, faculty who oversee student research need to be able to verify the integrity of their students' data collection.

An aspect of academic integrity to which nurse educators may have given less consideration is that of peer violations of academic integrity. Faculty, like students, need to adhere scrupulously to disciplinary standards for scholarship and to institutional policies related to grants, the conduct of research, institutional sponsorship, and external contracts. Faculty who serve as peer reviewers of manuscripts and grants must be meticulous in their protection of this information until it is officially made public. Faculty may discover their own intellectual property has been used without their permission; in such a situation the institutional legal department can be a helpful resource in determining how to respond (Martinson, Anderson, & deVries, 2005).

The human resources department or the academic affairs unit of an institution often publicizes standards of civility, policies related to employee behavior toward students and peers, and student behavior. These are likely to include policies related to discrimination, sexual harassment, and hate speech. Both lateral violence and faculty bullying of students are topics that have received considerable attention in the nursing education literature (Clark, 2008; Heinrich, 2007).

In recent years nurse educators have begun to address standards for the use of social media. Although some institutions attempt to forbid nursing students' use of social media, others have incorporated social media into education and patient care. For example, a simulated patient may have a Facebook page that provides a realistic means for a case study to unfold in real time. Or faculty may elicit succinct feedback from students on a particular issue using Twitter. It is important for nurse educators to be in dialogue about relevant policies with the educational institution as a whole and also with the clinical agencies with whom they affiliate. Some health care organizations are promoting patients' and providers' use of social media to reduce unnecessary health visits by providing timely answers to questions. Students need to appreciate their obligation to protect patients' personal information, including images that might include patients, and to understand they must conform to the rules of their practicum sites. This is a rapidly evolving issue in health care, and nurse educators may find the National Council of State Boards of Nursing's (2011) statement on the use of social media to be helpful.

Increasingly nursing educators encounter students and faculty with physical, mental health, or learning disabilities. The Americans with Disabilities Act mandates reasonable accommodation for students to meet learning objectives and for faculty to fulfill the demands of their employment (May, 2013). Faculty members need to know what their institution's policies and resources are related to accommodation of students and employees. Ultimately it is they who determine what constitutes reasonable accommodation related to nursing practice requirements, and they may benefit from consultation with such resources as the Association on Higher Education and Disability (2012) or the National Organization of Nurses with Disabilities (2013).

Nurse educators are increasingly likely to teach not only students who are immigrants or first-generation Americans, but also international students who are expected to return to their home countries. Academic departments establish criteria for international students that may include assessment of their English language ability as well as their academic background, proof of their licensure in their home country, a clinical practice requirement, and regulatory requirements such as criminal background checks and drug screening. Schools vary in requiring licensure in this country, and faculty need to weight that decision within the context of practicum requirements for a particular educational program. Effective work with international students requires some understanding of the educational and health care system in students' home countries, religious and cultural values, and behavioral norms, including family and gender roles. International students may bring their families, or they may leave their families, including young children, at home in their native country. Faculty must understand the requirements associated with students' visas related to study, travel, and employment. International students are likely to need support in areas such as locating housing, banking, transportation, coping with a new climate, and social connectedness to an extent exceeding most students' needs. Students may have had little or no experience with American educational norms such as multiple-choice examinations or scholarly writing consistent with format standards. It is important to identify resources in the institution, including other students, faculty, or staff from their countries, as well as community members who can help them adjust to and succeed in their new academic setting (Poyrazli & Grahame, 2007).

CONSIDER THE GOALS OF THE NURSING PROGRAM AND THE MISSION OF THE PARENT INSTITUTION WHEN PROPOSING CHANGE OR MANAGING ISSUES

Academic programs need to further the overall mission of the institution in which they reside. In colleges and universities, the academic nursing unit is likely to function with a higher degree of multidisciplinary collaboration than in a free-standing nursing or health professions educational institution. Undergraduate nursing programs in particular may be expected to incorporate a core common to all undergraduate students that aligns with the overall mission, heritage, and values of the institution. For example, a religiously affiliated college may have an unusually significant requirement in religious studies, philosophy, and ethics. All students in the institution, no matter their major, may be required to participate in an international immersion experience. There may be a service learning requirement in addition to the nursing practica. Students may need to fulfill requirements in writing, numeracy, cultural diversity, civics, fine arts, foreign languages, or even swimming. Faculty in baccalaureate as well as graduate programs in more research intensive environments may be urged to increase the opportunity for individual student research. It becomes a challenge for nurse educators to design academic programs that respond sufficiently to both institutional mission-driven as well as professional requirements. To keep the nursing program within a reasonable total of credits, faculty will find themselves debating how to trade old curriculum content for new additions. Nurse educators may be assisted in their work by the opportunity to participate in faculty development workshops that foster their appreciation of values that are central to their institution.

In terms of managing groups of faculty, nursing academic administrators are mindful of the expectations of an individual institution as they assign teaching and advise faculty members about time management in relation to the expectations of their appointments. In a teaching-focused institution there is a fairly high degree of consistency in how faculty members perceive their roles and how teaching assignments are distributed. Faculty might have time dedicated to their own clinical practice, and some faculty may be downloaded for administrative responsibilities, and other faculty members will support their own academic unit as well as the larger institution through committee work. But in general, faculty members in these organizations understand they are all there to implement the curriculum.

As institutions become more heavily focused on graduate education and particularly on research, the expectations become more diverse. Graduate faculty might have teaching assignments that include less direct clinical supervision or classroom instruction and more individual mentoring of students. Individual mentoring may not appear on teaching schedules, and their loads may appear to be much lighter than those of the undergraduate faculty. Faculty with research expectations may receive substantial teaching downloads at times, for instance, prior to tenure; this can seem unfair to nontenure track faculty or to older tenured faculty who did not have such an advantage when they were new faculty. Faculty with funding for research may be able to buy out most of their teaching time, but they will face expectations to mentor students or junior faculty in research and to produce and publish results within a specified time frame, which may also include writing the next grants to continue their work. Transparency about who is doing what and the expectations that all faculty face along with open dialogue for meeting the academic unit's goals can go a long way toward ameliorating perceptions of unfairness (Schuster & Finkelstein, 2006).

Academic administrators are increasingly focused on the generation of funds to support students financially, to support the costs of their more traditional programs, as well as to fund the expensive technology that is increasingly required to ensure students' competence, such as simulation labs. Fundraising may come from submission of grants for program development, facilities, or equipment; research grants that pay overhead to the school; solicitation of donations from alumni and philanthropists interested in nursing; and the development of profit-bearing academic and nonacademic programs. The number of new nontraditional programs such as accelerated second-degree programs or online RN-BSN and graduate programs have exploded in the past 20 years. These can be ways of reaching large numbers of students in a way that is highly cost-effective and profitable, even in nonprofit institutions (Ruth, 2006). Other types of programmatic outreach include continuing education, study tours, and education in health-related areas for other health professionals or for laypeople.

As institutions of higher learning face the decision of whether to join the institutions that are producing or using massive online open courses (MOOCs) or developing online programs, nursing units will be part of these discussions. MOOCs offer an opportunity to publicize widely what a school may be doing well, advertise their programs, and attract students from all over the world to enroll for credit (i.e., pay tuition). Online programs offer some of the same advantages. Opportunities such as this may be desirable for a school of nursing, but they also may be a drain on resources with little return. Still, nurse educators cannot ignore this trend.

Colleges and universities typically have institutional evaluation plans that examine outcomes related to every component of the organization, from, for example, its financial management to the quality of food in the dining hall, health and safety standards in the dormitories, compliance with National Collegiate Athletic Association rules, as well as each academic program. Institutional accountability mandates that schools assess how well they are meeting the needs of students in all respects, particularly given the high cost of higher education. In addition, a school must be responsive to standards from government and professional organizations governing every aspect of its operations. Periodically schools will draw on their evaluation data as they prepare self-studies for accreditation. Ideally the massive quantity of data that are collected each year across a college or university is used not only for the purpose of reporting, but also for continuous improvement and mapping progress in fulfilling the organization's strategic plan (Allen, 2004).

A well-informed faculty member understands that this activity is ongoing and will at times be invited to participate in it. One routine way that faculty engage with institutional evaluation plans is their participation in the evaluation of teaching by students and by their peers and administrators. Institutions vary in the extent to which these evaluations are made public within the organization. Another way is through periodic evaluations of overall faculty performance, including the three components of the faculty role—teaching, scholarship, and service—in the balance particular to the institution and the faculty member's appointment. Finally, nurse educators may serve on committees related to self-studies in their own academic unit or across the institution. Institutions aggregate data related to faculty performance (e.g., numbers of credits and students taught, publications, grants, grant dollars, committees, and professional offices), and this information may be used as a basis for recommendations about increasing cost-effectiveness of academic programs.

One challenge for nursing faculty is that clinical practice may or may not be regarded by the institution as a component of the faculty role. In some institutions nurse faculty practice is regarded as competitive with full-time employment by the institution, and they may need to apply for special permission to engage in it, although some nursing education administrators have been successful in negotiating recognition for faculty practice. This can be a particularly challenging dilemma for faculty members whose certifications require a significant amount of clinical practice and who are employed to teach in a track that requires them to maintain certification (Paskiewicz, 2003). In some institutions, faculty members who teach in advanced practice programs are ineligible for the tenure track because of their substantial practice requirements.

Institutions of higher education often have an interest in the development of the student as a whole person. Faculty members may be called on to interact with students in capacities beyond formal teaching and advising, and they may find it enlightening as well as rewarding to interact with students outside the nursing major. Opportunities may involve such activities as co-curricular learning interactions, participation in volunteer service, or faculty sponsorship of a student organization or activity. Students gain from the opportunity to relate to faculty outside their formal roles, and these can be ways to encourage students in all disciplines to consider careers in higher education.

PARTICIPATE ON INSTITUTIONAL AND DEPARTMENTAL COMMITTEES

Nurse educators are well served to know how the nursing unit fits into the overall organizational chart of the institution as well as who are the top level administrators and members of the board of trustees. It is strategic to know what some of the important accomplishments are in various academic and nonacademic units, as faculty members represent their institutions as a whole in the local community and through their professional activities and will be asked about these matters.

There are opportunities throughout the year in most educational institutions to interact with institutional leaders as well as colleagues at all levels from across the institution. This is important for several reasons. Research indicates that women faculty members tend to give less time and attention to business-related social interactions, to the detriment of their advancement in the college or university (White, 2005). It can be extremely important when a faculty member seeks tenure or promotion to be known by deans, tenure committee members, and administrators who will be making the decision on their behalf. Moreover, when a nursing faculty member is engaged in a matter that relates to, or requires assistance from, others in the system (e.g., seeking to change the way a nonnursing course in the nursing curriculum is being taught), it is invaluable to have relationships with these people prior to seeking their help. Interactions with academic colleagues throughout the institution may lead to ideas for interprofessional courses, service learning activities, or research projects. Moreover, it is extremely enlightening to learn about the organization through the eyes of people outside of one's own discipline. For some institutional activities, attendance is mandatory, and by all means faculty members must be attentive to those expectations; but even if they are not, it is wise to participate.

As mentioned previously, faculty at some institutions are members of organized labor units and engage in collective bargaining related to the terms of their contracts. Faculty members who are at a unionized institution need to understand what it means professionally to join or not join the union, as well as the issues under discussion and the political costs and benefits of being actively engaged in advocacy related to their contracts at various stages of their careers. Specifically, it may be unwise for a tenure-track faculty member to run for office in the collective bargaining unit, although after tenure, a faculty member can offer the perspective of time in the institution with little risk.

Most higher education institutions have a structure for faculty governance, such as a faculty senate, and this is a way for faculty members to be represented on major committees of the institution. These can include, for example, the committee for tenure and promotion, committees related to salary and benefits, search committees for administrative positions, committees related to self-studies of areas within the institution or the institution as a whole, administrator evaluation committees, athletic department oversight, strategic planning committees, and the board of trustees or committees of the board. Some positions may be elected, although most are appointed or voluntary. These venues provide important means for the faculty to have a voice in the future direction of the institution. Also, the nursing faculty need to be part of institutional decisions that affect their educational programs. In addition, participation in governance provides important leadership development opportunities for faculty members, and these experiences are invaluable to nurse educators who aspire to assume a leadership role within the nursing education unit. Although service on committees of the institution is important in the career of a nurse educator, it is also very important to balance one's time appropriately between the teaching, scholarship, and service expectations of one's particular institution and employment agreement.

SUMMARY

- Nursing education programs are located in a variety of types of institutions that may be focused on nursing, or health profession schools affiliated with a health system, or colleges and universities that offer a variety of degrees in many disciplines.
- Nurse educators need to be aware of the specific heritage and mission of their institution and how the nursing program supports it.
- Nurse educators need to be conversant with accreditation standards to which their program and institution adhere as they continually evaluate program quality and as they revise or expand program offerings.
- Nurse educators need to understand the terms of their employment agreement in relation to the balance of their total responsibilities for teaching, scholarship, and service; the onsite schedule; clinical practice; and annual contracted service.
- The communities of interest to which a nursing program needs to respond include students, alumni, employers, the institution as a whole, governmental and professional regulatory agencies, donors, and the community.
- Particular student populations have specific needs, and societal trends or historical events raise awareness of issues to which educational programs need to respond.
- Faculty need to understand the fiscal profile of their academic unit within the context of the institution.
- Nurse educators serve their programs by representing them through faculty self-governance and on institutional committees that determine policy and broadly evaluate the organization's function and outcomes.

Practice Test Questions

1. Which of the following does *not* accurately describe a type of institution in which academic nursing programs are found?
   A. Research intensive university
   B. Health sciences school affiliated with a health system
   C. Religious seminary
   D. Proprietary college

2. The Institution of Medicine's *Future of Nursing* report of 2010 recommended that:
   A. All advanced practice nurses be prepared as doctors of nursing practice starting in 2020
   B. All associate degree programs transition to baccalaureate programs by 2020
   C. Eighty percent of baccalaureate prepared nurses earn master's degrees by 2020
   D. Eighty percent of all nurses be prepared at a baccalaureate or higher degree level by 2020

3. The traditional academic role in an institution of higher education is a balance among:
   A. Teaching, scholarship, and service
   B. Clinical practice, teaching, and administration
   C. Teaching, evaluation, and service
   D. Teaching, grant writing, and research

4. A nursing professor stated in his medical-surgical nursing class that in a situation of total physical immobility, he would not want life-prolonging interventions. A student complained to the department chair that her religious values were disparaged by the professor. The department chair's best response would be:
   A. No response, as the faculty member had a right to offer this comment in class
   B. To schedule a disciplinary meeting with the faculty member for violating the student's religious freedom
   C. To prohibit nursing faculty from commenting on their personal preferences in health care
   D. To refer the situation to the institution's chief officer for academic affairs

5. A major principle behind the promotion of interprofessional education is:
   A. It is personally enriching for students to learn in groups of diverse majors
   B. Nurses will be less likely to use jargon if they experience interprofessional education
   C. Interprofessional education promotes communication strategies that improve patient safety
   D. Significant funding for nursing education is available for interprofessional education

References

Allen, M. J. (2004). *Assessing academic programs in higher education*. Bolton, MA: Anker.

American Association of University Professors (AAUP). (2013). Mission & description. Retrieved from http://www.aaup.org/about/mission-description

American Nurses Association. (2013). ANA supports joining forces. Retrieved from http://nursingworld.org/MainMenuCategories/ThePracticeof ProfessionalNursing/Improving-Your-Practice/ ANA-Supports-Joining-Forces/default.aspx

Anonymous. (1939). Accrediting moves forward. *American Journal of Nursing, 39*(6), 647–648.

Anonymous. (2012, December 1). Not what it used to be. The Economist. Retrieved from http://www.economist.com/news/united-states/21567373-american-universities-represent-declining-value-money-their-students-not-what-it

Association on Higher Education and Disability. (2012). Welcome to AHEAD! Retrieved from http://www.ahead.org/

Baer, E. D. (2012). Key ideas in nursing's first century. *American Journal of Nursing, 112*(5), 48–55.

Benson, A. (2013). Labor market trends among registered nurses: 2008–2011. Policy, politics and nursing practice. Retrieved from http://intl-ppn.sagepub.com/content/early/2013/04/29/15271544134818 10.full.pdf+html

Brown, E. L. (1948). *Nursing for the future*. New York: Russell Sage Foundation.

Carnegie Foundation for the Advancement of Teaching. (2013). The Carnegie classification of institutions of higher education. Retrieved from http://classifications.carnegiefoundation.org/

Clark, C. M. (2008). Student voices on faculty incivility in nursing education: A conceptual model. *Nursing Education Perspectives, 29*(5), 284–289.

Commission on Collegiate Nursing Education (CCNE). (2013). CCNE standards & professional nursing guidelines. Retrieved from http://www.aacn.nche.edu/ccne-accreditation/standards-procedures-resources/baccalaureate-graduate/standards

Committee for the Study of Nursing Education. (1923). *Nursing and nursing education in the United States*. New York: Macmillan.

Council for Higher Education Accreditation. (2013). Regional accrediting organizations 2012–2013. Retrieved from http://www.chea.org/Directories/regional.asp

Delbanco, A. (2012). *College: What it was, is, and should be*. Princeton, NJ: Princeton University Press.

Evaluating Innovations in Nursing Education. (2013). Robert Wood Johnson Foundation. Retrieved from http://www.evaluatinginnovationsinnursing.org/

Health Resources and Services Administration (HRSA). (2013). *The US nursing workforce: Trends in supply and education*. Washington, DC: U.S. Department of Health and Human Services. Retrieved from http://bhpr.hrsa.gov/healthworkforce/reports/nursing-workforce/index.html

Heinrich, K. (2007). Joy stealing: 10 mean games faculty play and how to stop the gaming. *Nurse Educator, 32*(1), 34–38.

Institute of Medicine (IOM). (2010). *The future of nursing: Leading change, advancing health*. Washington, DC: National Academies Press.

Institute of Medicine (IOM). (1999). *To err is human: Building a safer health system*. Washington, DC: National Academies Press.

International Council of Nurses. (2013). About ICN. Retrieved from http://icn-apnetwork.org/

Larson, E. (2012). New rules for the game: Interdisciplinary education for health professionals. *Nursing Outlook, 60*, 264–271.

Levine, H., & Scorsone, E. (2011). The great recession's institutional change in the public employment relationships: implications for state and local governments. *State and Local Government Review, 43*(3), 208–214.

Martinson, B. C., Anderson, M. S., & deVries, R. (2005). Scientists behaving badly. *Nature, 435*, 737–738.

May, K. (2013). Assessing faculty knowledge of disability-related law and providing academic accommodation. Unpublished PhD Dissertation. Villanova University College of Nursing, Villanova, PA.

Montag, M. (1959). *Community college education for nursing*. New York: McGraw-Hill.

National Council of State Boards of Nursing. (2011). White paper: A nurse's guide to the use of social media. Retrieved from https://www.ncsbn.org/Social_media_guidelines.pdf

National League for Nursing Accreditation Commission (NLNAC). (2013a). Search for NLNAC accredited programs. Retrieved from http://www.nlnac.org/forms/directory_search.htm

National League for Nursing Accreditation Commission (NLNAC). (2013b). 2013 NLNAC standards and criteria. Retrieved from http://www.nlnac.org/manuals/SC2013.htm

National League for Nursing Certification Commission Certification Test Development Committee. (2012). *The scope of practice for academic nurse educators*. New York: National League for Nursing.

National League of Nursing Education. (1937). *Curriculum guide for schools of nursing*. New York: National League of Nursing Education.

National Organization of Nurses with Disabilities. (2013). Questions and answers about health care workers and the Americans with Disabilities Act. Retrieved from http://www.nond.org/

Paskiewicz, L. A. (2003). Clinical practice: an emphasis strategy for promotion and tenure. *Nursing Forum, 38*(4), 21–26.

Poyrazli, S., & Grahame, K. M. (2007). Barriers to adjustment needs of international students within a semi-urban campus community. *Journal of Instructional Psychology, 34*(1), 28–45.

Riley, N. S. (2011). *The faculty lounges and other reasons why you won't get the college education you paid for*. Chicago: Ivan R. Dee.

Ruth, S. R. (2006, January 1). E-learning—a financial and strategic perspective. Educause Review Online. Retrieved from http://www.educause.edu/ero/article/e-learning%E2%80%94-financial-and-strategic-perspective

Schuster, J. H., & Finkelstein, M. J. (2006). *The American faculty: The restructuring of academic work and careers.* Baltimore: Johns Hopkins University Press.

Sigma Theta Tau International. (2013). STTI's global initiatives. Retrieved from http://www.nursingsociety.org/GlobalAction/Initiatives/Pages/building_global.aspx

Szabo, A., & Underwood, J. (2004). Cybercheats: Is information and communication technology fueling academic dishonesty? *Active Learning in Higher Education, 5*(2), 180–199.

U.S. Department of Education (DOE). (2013). The database of accredited postsecondary institutions and programs. Retrieved from http://ope.ed.gov/accreditation/

U.S. Department of Health and Human Services. (2013). Transform health care. Retrieved from http://www.hhs.gov/secretary/about/transform.html

White, J. S. (2005). Pipeline to pathways: New directions for improving the status of women campus. *Liberal Education, 91*(1), 22–27.

Guide to Educational Learning Theories

Theory	Principles	Application to Learning
Behaviorism	Learning is the result of changes in behavior. Learning is reinforced by response. Stimuli and responses are connected. Prior experience (reinforcements/punishments) determines behaviors. Conditioning determines how individuals respond to a learning situation, as well as the rate at which individuals respond. Theorists: Watson, Skinner, Thorndike	Learning is shaped by others, and students are not held to be individually responsible for their learning. The teacher and environment hold responsibility for learning. Students are motivated by extrinsic rewards. Use of behavioral course objectives is rooted in behaviorism. Examples of teaching methods: learning contracts and programmed instruction modules.
Cognitivism (Information Processing Theories)	Emphasizes the person's cognitive or thinking processes. Views the learner as more active in the learning process than behaviorism. Learning involves internal processes such as memory, perception, problem solving, reasoning and concept formation. To acquire information that can be retrieved later, connections to other ideas, prior knowledge, and experience and emotions are necessary. Changes in the learner are an indication of change in cognition. Control for learning is less focused on the environment (behaviorism) and more focused on the learner's mental engagement. Theorists: Brunner, Ausubel, Gagne	Relating incoming information to previously learned information makes it more memorable. The way information is presented to the learner can facilitate and detract from learning. The individual needs to be active in creating a structured network of information (i.e., concept map, comparing ideas, rehearsal, study cards). Examples of teaching methods: group projects, role playing, computerized simulations, teaching foundational facts before higher levels of knowledge.
Social Learning Theory	Hybrid of behaviorist and cognitivist perspectives. Learner and environment are in a reciprocal relationship in which each influences the other. Self-efficacy of one's personal ability and one's sense of self-determination are influential to learning. Modeling or learning through observation is essential. Theorist: Bandura	Learning occurs from passive as well as deliberate observation of behavior. Reflection on the negative consequences of behavior influences limited repetition of the behavior. Teaching methods: self-evaluation of learning, observation of best practices, mastery experiences.

(continued on page 142)

Theory	Principles	Application to Learning
Constructivism	Learning occurs through experience. Learning is actively constructed by the learner and involves actions and reflection of prior experiences to derive meaning. The teaching method is not the determining factor; the active process that the learner uses is key. Learning should include integrating subject matter through application to everyday life. Direct contrast to the passive learning of behaviorism. Learning involves active problem solving, perception, values, and meaning. Theorists: Dewey, Piaget	Students take an active role in learning and construct knowledge out of their own experiences. Peer influences make a difference in learning engagement. It is essential to be able to suspend belief and not be worried about peer pressure to engage in learning. Learners need to motivate from within to have a transformative experience. Examples of teaching methods: making comparisons and associations with previous knowledge, reflective logs, debate.
Humanism	Individuals act with intentionality based on values and needs. Learning is based on human generation of knowledge, meaning, and ultimately expertise through interpersonal and intrapersonal intelligence. The learning goal is to become self-actualized with intrinsic motivation toward accomplishment. The learner is able to adapt prior knowledge to new experiences. Person-centered learning addresses the learner's intellect, social skills, and feelings or intuitions. Theorists: Rogers, Maslow, Freire, Glasser	Acquisition, development, and integration of knowledge occur through strategy, personal interpretation, evaluation, reasoning, and decision making. The educator's role is to encourage and enable the learner, by providing access to appropriate resources without obtrusive interference. The learning goal is high-order learning of reasoning, abstract analysis, and development of expertise. Teaching methods: classrooms that are student-centered where teachers and students express ideas and perspectives, personal interactions with students that promote positive regard and increase self-esteem.

References

All, A. C., Huycke, L.I., Fisher, M. J. (2003). Instructional tools for nursing education: Concept maps. *Nursing Education Perspectives, 34,* 311–317.

Bandura, A. (1977). *Social learning theory.* Englewood Cliffs, NJ: Prentice Hall.

Bruner, J. (1964). The course of cognitive growth. *American Psychologst, 19,* 1–15.

Dewey, J. (1910/1997). *How we think.* Mineola, NY: Dover.

Gagne, R.M., Wager, W. W., Golas, K.C., Keller, J. M. (2005). *Principles of instructional design* (5th ed.). Belmont, CA: Thomas/Wadsworth Publishing.

Hmelo-Silver, C. (2004). Problem-based learning. What and how do students learn? *Educational Psychology Review 16*(3), 235–266.

Kuiper, R. and Pesut, D. (2004). Promoting cognitive and metacognitive relective reasoning skills in nursing practice: Self-regulated learning theory. *Journal of Advanced Nursing, 45*(4), 381–391.

Maslow, A. H. (1968). *Toward a psychology of being* (2nd ed.). New York: Van Nostrand.

Rogers, C., & Freiberg, H. J. (1994). *Freedome to learn* (3rd ed.). New York: Charles Merrill.

Slavin, R. E. (2006). *Educational psychology: Theory and practice.* New York: Pearson.

Schunk, D. H. (2012). *Learning theories: An educational perspective* (6th ed.). New York: Pearson.

Utley, R. (2011). *Theory and research for academic nurse educators.* Sudbury, MA: Jonas and Bartlett Publishers.

Answers to Practice Test Questions

Chapter 1

1. Answer: D

Rationale: Simulation requires the learner to choose an action and see the consequences in a safe environment; most students require active engagement rather than passive observation. Students report being bored when they just sit and watch other students perform.

2. Answer: B

Rationale: The content is ever expanding and it is difficult to know all the content. Plus, it changes with the addition of new research. Students need to learn how to use technology to find the most current evidence to support their care of patients. Unfortunately, three-quarters of all programs have yet to create this course.

3. Answer: A

Rationale: Using structured critical thinking terminology will frequently help students gain experience and confidence in using critical thinking for actual cases. The other options offer passive learning or do not provide immediate feedback to students regarding their thinking.

4. Answer: C

Rationale: Helping students realize that when teams are diverse, teams are stronger, and there are many examples of diversity. By asking students to work with other students with different learning styles from their own, students can become more aware of their own and others' learning styles.

5. Answer: B

Rationale: Providing quality feedback in a positive way impacts all learners. When they see the teacher is supportive and creates a safe environment to learn and practice and make mistakes, they are more willing to try. Trying allows students to succeed. Excellent teachers give feedback in a positive way rather than a negative way.

6. Answer: D

Rationale: Clinical judgment is supported when students are asked to prioritize care for multiple clients and recognize changing conditions. Helping students prioritize facilitates the development of clinical judgment, a marker of an expert nurse.

7. Answer: D

Rationale: These students, being digital natives and great multitaskers, have a hard time being still and having to focus on a lecture. By engaging them in activity, and using technology, they will learn to apply the material being taught.

8. Answer: A

Rationale: Research shows that enthusiasm in teaching engages students and inspires them to achieve more. Students think excellent educators show enthusiasm, passion, love, and joy and this carries over to the students' studies.

9. Answer: C

Rationale: Asking students to sit quietly during a lecture and listen is difficult for these multitaskers, who have grown up with technology. Rather than having them put away technology, ask them to bring it out and use it for active learning. Helping them learn how to use technology for learning will help them develop lifelong habits of critical thinking and independent searching for information.

10. Answer: B

Rationale: Collegiality allows for equality in expressing opinions; it also allows for diversity of thought. When faculty realize all have the same goal but can arrive at the goal from different paths, this takes the emotion out of the decision and the group can remain collegial—mutual respect, equal partners.

Chapter 2

1. Answer: A

Rationale: B, C, and D are not conducive to adult learning. It is important for the nurse educator to collaborate with adult learners to identify learning needs and develop learning experiences to meet those needs. In general, adult learners tend to be more self-directed and require less structure to meet learning outcomes.

2. Answer: C

Rationale: This assignment requires students to relate together information for a complex medical patient, which requires a high level of thinking. Using a concept map, students express the concept and its relationship to other elements in a visual format. The map enables students to think critically, synthesize and organize information, and demonstrate relationships. Algorithms are maps that break decision-making issues into step-by-step procedures that lead to yes/no answers or actions. They do not demonstrate relationships, but are best used to teach the steps of a complex procedure. The one-minute paper is best used to assess the comprehension of major course concepts, but would lack the depth to analyze a complex situation. Simulation is best to evaluate skills in a more authentic environment, but would not meet this objective.

3. Answer: C

Rationale: To best master a psychomotor skill, the student should practice consistently over time. Through consistent repetition the nurse internalizes a psychomotor skill. Performance of the skill becomes natural and precise. The instructor is student oriented and fosters development. With a complex skill, the instructor should allow time for remediation and coach the student until he or she is proficient in this skill. The other strategies, paper and reflection in a journal or orally, would not be appropriate for a manual skill.

4. Answer: D

Rationale: Interaction between the teacher and students is the most important factor to engage students with the material to be studied and to facilitate their learning with any of the learning styles.

5. Answer: C

Rationale: The affective domain of learning reflects the student's growth in feelings or emotional areas. The student demonstrates belief in the value of an individual. This ranges from simple acceptance to the more complex state of commitment.

6. Answer: D

Rationale: Difficulties experienced by ESL students are frequently the result of language issues. Research suggests that pairing ESL students with native English speakers who can coach them in proper use and understanding of English helps improve overall language proficiency.

7. Answer: B

Rationale: Kinesthetic learners excel when experiencing the world through tactile sensation and movement. Providing opportunities to practice skills or play with equipment maximizes their learning.

8. Answer: A

Rationale: How students take in knowledge and make sense of it is key to experiential learning, which Kolb considers a requirement for adaptation. Thus, in order to learn, new information is constantly compared with what is known from previous experience. Ultimately, either the previous experiences or the new knowledge is seen in a new light, as the learner adapts beliefs, values, and understanding.

9. Answer: D

Rationale: Although A, B, and C are all important, the nurse educator ultimately has the responsibility to patient safety. Evidence is mounting that suggests that disruptive behavior and incivility in the workplace jeopardize patient safety. Thus, it is more and more essential that students and new graduates display appropriate relational skills.

10. Answer: B

Rationale: Students must self-disclose disabilities and formally request accommodation under the ADA. Reasonable accommodations must be offered and are considered in the context of a program's resources. Although accommodations may include adjusting clinical experiences or modifying examinations, ultimately the student must successfully achieve the established program objectives.

Chapter 3

1. Answer: C

Rationale: Guiding questions in summative evaluation include: Were behavioral objectives met? Did the individual(s) learn? Options A and B assess learning during one specific time and are not summative, and D is program evaluation.

2. Answer: B

Rationale: Options A, C, and D are examples of norm-referenced interpretation. Criterion-referenced interpretation of data is typically used in competency-based models to assess achievement of competence in, or mastery of, specified learning outcomes.

3. Answer: B

Rationale: Comparing a student's work to another's is an example of norm referencing. Option A, criterion referencing, assesses student work based on preset standards or criteria. C and D are forms of evaluation and are not related to grading on a curve.

4. Answer: C

Rationale: If there are several faculty members teaching a course and responsible for a group of students in that course, interrater reliability must be established to maintain consistency, eliminate bias, and ensure fairness for all students in the class.

5. Answer: D

Rationale: A range greater than 30 indicates discrimination between low-scoring and high-scoring students. For option A, reliability is high, for B, the analysis indicates that the higher scoring students answered the item correctly, and for C, the acceptable range for difficulty is greater than 30 percent.

6. Answer: A

Rationale: The difficulty value (p value) indicates the percentage of students who selected the correct answer. B is incorrect as a negative PBCC indicates that low-scoring students selected this answer more than high-scoring students. C is incorrect as more high-scoring students selected this answer. D is incorrect as the overall PBCC of 0.09 does not discriminate at greater than 0.20, the desired range.

7. Answer: A

Rationale: B, C, and D are not valid purposes of an item analysis.

8. Answer: A

Rationale: The response is asking the student to recall what is meant by contact precautions. Options B, C, and D require higher-level thinking in the Bloom's taxonomy range.

9. Answer: C

Rationale: Option A is recall, B is comprehension, and D is application.

Chapter 4

1. Answer: B

Rationale: The language of the competency must reflect a continued state of development of the nursing student. Development may take the form of increasing complexity, differentiation, delineation, or sophistication. Each competency leads to the eventual development of a competent care provider.

2. Answer: A

Rationale: The first step in developing a curriculum is to determine the desired characteristics of the new graduates. The current curriculum is 25 years old, so the theoretical framework for that curriculum is outdated. C and D are tasks to be completed but come later in the curriculum revision process.

3. Answer: D

Rationale: Course content must build on that of prerequisite nursing courses. Option A is incorrect because the two nursing programs may be structured differently. B is incorrect because the textbook is a reference but not the guide to curriculum; not all information in the textbook may be designated important information to be taught. Although faculty are expert nurses, personal opinion may guide decisions, leading to content that is taught for the wrong reasons; therefore, C is not the correct answer.

4. Answer: B

Rationale: B provides the overall purpose of the program assessment plan. Options A, C, and D are addressed in an assessment plan, but they do not represent the overall purpose of a program assessment plan.

5. Answer: A

Rationale: Option A provides an open-ended question that specifically addresses what nurses do in the current health care environment. This is important information for developing a current curriculum. B might yield institution-specific information that may not be generalized for other institutions. C elicits a yes/no answer that does not provide useful information. D is not related to the purpose of the program.

Chapter 5

1. Answer: A

Rationale: Completing a self-assessment with a well-developed rubric helps identify learning needs and further learning plans as one's own.

2. Answer: A

Professional service is typically considered volunteer work at the program, university, or professional organizational level. Extending paid clinical hours would typically not be considered extending service.

3. Answer: D

Rationale: Balancing involves combining roles and working collaboratively with team members. Mentoring includes assisting an individual to find a "better way" to accomplish scholarly activities.

4. Answer: C

Rationale: Socialization is about meeting with and learning from various team members about resources and opportunities, rather than being totally "I" focused.

5. Answer: B

Rationale: Proactive strategies for helping students understand the concept of academic integrity are best in promoting student professional behaviors.

6. Answer: D

Rationale: The student handbook provides basic faculty guidance about appropriate reactive strategies when a student demonstrates a problem behavior. Your response must be consistent with the policies set forth in the student handbook.

7. Answer: C

Rationale: Success in professional development involves self-directed learner interest and commitment. Enrollment in a nursing practice doctorate program may be reasonable for this faculty if his interests are consistent with his administrator's, but that is not indicated in the question.

8. Answer: B

Rationale: Career success is typically guided by a good match on interests with the organization's mission as well as strong program orientation opportunities. At this point the faculty candidate should already have gained information about the program orientation and the fit between the faculty's interests and those of the organization.

Chapter 6

1. Answer: C

Rationale: Leaders focus on long-term goals, articulate goals that arise from their passion for excellence, collaborate with followers, and have power because of what they know. In contrast, mangers focus on task accomplishment, articulate goals that are formulated by the organization, direct subordinates in their work, and have power because of their formal position of authority in the organization.

2. Answer: B

Rationale: Surveying faculty about the need for change is not necessarily an indication of an individual's cultural sensitivity, nor is it merely attending lectures on diversity. Although asking representatives from various "subgroups" to review a proposal for change might suggest a desire to obtain the perspectives of various groups, those "subgroups" may not necessarily have any relation to cultural diversity, and the feedback from them may not be incorporated. By acknowledging that each individual who will participate in the change process is unique and likely to react to and engage with the process in different ways because of that uniqueness, the nursing education leader role models cultural sensitivity.

3. Answer: B

Rationale: Readiness for change can best be evaluated by gaining an understanding of the extent and nature of change recently experienced by the group, as well as understanding the degree to which administration supports a proposed change. If members of a group have been involved in extensive change over a lengthy period of time, if past experiences with change have been negative, or if individuals perceive that administration is not supportive of a proposed change—and may, indeed, say the change cannot be implemented—their willingness to participate in yet another major change is likely to be quite limited. Reviewing evaluations of a curriculum development presentation may provide information about the extent to which the presentation helped faculty understand curriculum design, but it does not necessarily give any indication of their readiness to undertake a major curriculum change. Similarly, learning about the nursing practice experiences of faculty is not helpful in determining their readiness to engage in curriculum revision work. And while comments made at a meeting may be a "clue" to the individual attempting to lead the curriculum change that faculty are not aligned with the goals of the change, such information is not indicative of their readiness for transformative change in the curriculum.

4. Answer: C

Rationale: A nursing education leader can demonstrate her or his passion for new ideas and articulate a vision of a more effective, engaging, meaningful educational experience for students by explicating a radically different approach to course design and implementation. Such a vision is needed to help colleagues consider and, indeed, move to create a better program. When such a vision evolves from a synthesis of research findings and recommendations from experts in the field, one can be confident that it defines a preferred future, one that is desirable and is an improvement over what now exists. Although it might be important to consider workload implications, relationships with clinical partners, and program evaluation standards when implementing educational change, attention to such details is relevant only after the vision of a preferred future is articulated, as was done by the nursing education leader in this example.

5. Answer: A

Rationale: Effective leaders help others see a better way to do things and motivate those individuals to join in making those things happen. In other words, they clearly articulate a vision and motivate others to help realize it. Change and innovation will not necessarily occur because the individual advocating for them holds a position of authority in an organization, is tenured, holds the rank of professor, chairs a committee, or outlines tasks to be done and timelines to be achieved. Such circumstances may very well position an individual to have greater influence in an organization, but they do not provide any assurance that others in the organization will be willing to invest the time and energy needed to create change and implement innovative approaches to teaching, assessment, curriculum design, new faculty orientation, and so on.

6. Answer: D

Rationale: Effective followers think critically, challenge ideas, question the status quo, do not follow blindly, are not "stuck" in the present, and do more than merely listen. They participate actively and collaborate with the leader to "make things happen."

7. Answer: C

Rationale: Typically, it is the dean, chair, or director who acts as the spokesperson for the school within the parent institution, although this may be delegated to individual faculty in certain circumstances. When such a role is delegated, however, the representing faculty member is expected to convey the perspectives of the dean or director. Although faculty may be asked to provide input as the school's budget or strategic plan is being developed, responsibility for making final decisions about the budget and strategic plan and overseeing their implementation rests with the individual in the designated position of authority. Any faculty member (including the dean or chair) who is providing leadership within the school may, however, help members of the faculty engage in evidence-based teaching practices. Indeed, providing such help may be a strategy implemented by the nursing education leader to facilitate change on a larger scale.

8. Answer: A

Rationale: The nurse educator who accepts an invitation or nomination to have her or his name placed on a ballot for election to office in a national organization is exhibiting leadership and a desire to influence the future direction of that organization. Even if the individual is not elected to office, the fact that she or he took the risk, was viewed as someone with ideas or perspectives to offer that could benefit the organization, and expressed a willingness to work in a larger forum to create change all suggest qualities of a leader. Although maintaining a practice is laudable, it is not necessarily an indication of leadership or a willingness to facilitate change. Likewise, talking with students about the importance of scholarly work and professional involvement is valuable, but it does not necessarily mean that the faculty member actually takes on such responsibilities her- or himself. Finally, leaders strive for excellence and do not settle for mediocrity or the status quo; therefore, advocating to keep things as they are simply because there are no major negative outcomes is not characteristic of a leader or change agent.

9. Answer: D

Rationale: Coordinating a health fair for members of the institutional community best demonstrates leadership, clearly reflects the professional expertise of nurses, and serves to enhance the visibility of nursing within and its contributions to the parent institution. Serving as chair of a committee within the school at best reflects leadership within that limited community but does little to enhance the visibility of nursing at the institutional level. Volunteering at a local clinic, on the other hand, does enhance the visibility of nursing, but it is within the community rather than in the parent institution. Merely attending any kind of meeting does not indicate leadership, and while it is likely to be noted that "nursing has a representative" at the faculty senate meeting, lack of active involvement in those meetings will not serve to enhance the visibility of nursing within the institution.

10. Answer: B

Rationale: Lewin's change theory outlines three stages: unfreezing, moving, and refreezing. There is no separate data-gathering stage, although relevant data will need to be gathered during the unfreezing stage. In that first stage, participants explore the need for change, discuss the implications of the change, begin to appreciate the effort that will be involved to implement and sustain the change, and realize how they will need to change once the new approach is in place. All of this, understandably, makes many participants anxious and fearful; as a result, they may resist efforts to move toward making changes. Although financial support may be lacking as the change is put into place, and although some members of the group may try to sabotage or undermine the change once it has been implemented and is being integrated into "the new normal," these are not concerns facing the leader at the beginning of the change process.

Chapter 7

1. Answer: A

Rationale: Option A best describes the scholarship of discovery. B is consistent with the scholarship of integration. C describes the scholarship of teaching. D describes the scholarship of application.

2. Answer: D

Rationale: The scholarship of discovery encompasses original research or discovery of new knowledge. It is the foundation of the other three scholarships. Option A is an example of the scholarship of teaching, B is an example of the scholarship of application, and C is an example of the scholarship of teaching.

3. Answer: C

Rationale: Faculty should share their teaching expertise with their colleagues through publication and presentation of their innovative teaching methods and the outcomes of working with students.

4. Answer: A

Rationale: Leadership positions in professional organizations and on community or national panels and boards are considered scholarship of application.

5. Answer: B

Rationale: The rigor expected for scholarship of application is as high as that for other aspects. Although service expected of citizens is laudable, to constitute the scholarship of application the work must relate to the faculty member's expertise, be evaluated, and lead to new insights.

6. Answer: B

Rationale: Option A is important, but it would not constitute evidence-based teaching unless the innovation was evaluated; C is what many faculty members do, but it is not evidence-based teaching; D is one constraint noted to evidence-based teaching, but time would need to be negotiated well before the dossier is being prepared.

7. Answer: D

Rationale: Option A could be included if the syllabi were shared and demonstrated the evolution of teaching expertise, but standing alone would not demonstrate sharing of teaching expertise. B and C similarly would not demonstrate sharing of expertise, unless specific illustrations were included.

8. Answer: A

Rationale: It is the obligation of faculty members to ensure that students demonstrate behaviors consistent with professional codes of ethics and client autonomy or self-determination is included in the American Nurses Association (2010) "Code for Nurses." B is not correct, since the faculty member did not ask the student to avoid sharing his beliefs. C is incorrect; it would not be correct to ask a student to change his religious beliefs. D is not correct, although client autonomy must also be respected if he or she is being asked to participate in research.

9. Answer: C

Rationale: Option A is not the best answer, because research requires institutional review board (IRB) approval for protection of human subjects. Some educational evaluation projects may not require this review, but it is still a recommended practice to protect student interests. B is not correct, because payment could be construed as coercive. The IRB may approve small incentives, but review by this external group best protects student interests. D is not correct, because student interests supersede the value of the information.

Chapter 8
1. Answer: C

Rationale: Schools of nursing may be in free-standing nursing or health professions institutions associated with health systems or in colleges and universities. They can be public, private, or private religious; and they may be online or on physical campuses.

2. Answer: D

Rationale: The educational recommendations of the IOM's "Future of Nursing" report (2010) include the recommendation that 80 percent of all nurses be prepared at a baccalaureate or higher degree level by 2020.

3. Answer: A

Rationale: The traditional three facets of the faculty role are teaching, scholarship, and service; the percentage of emphasis on each varies according to the type of institution in which a nurse educator is teaching and the nurse educator's employment contract.

4. Answer: A

Rationale: The principle of academic freedom recognizes the expertise of faculty members within their content area as well as their right to choose teaching–learning strategies.

5. Answer: C

Rationale: Interprofessional education has grown in emphasis to better prepare health professionals to communicate respectfully and in a timely manner about potential threats to patient safety freely and without risk.

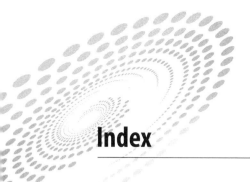

Index

Note: Page number followed by *f*, *b*, and *t* indicates figure, box, and table respectively.